Management of Benign and Malignant Pleural Effusions

Editor

CLIFF K.C. CHOONG

THORACIC SURGERY CLINICS

www.thoracic.theclinics.com

Consulting Editor
M. BLAIR MARSHALL

February 2013 • Volume 23 • Number 1

ELSEVIER

1600 John F. Kennedy Boulevard • Suite 1800 • Philadelphia, Pennsylvania, 19103-2899

http://www.theclinics.com

THORACIC SURGERY CLINICS Volume 23, Number 1
February 2013 ISSN 1547-4127, ISBN-13: 978-1-4557-7339-8

Editor: Jessica McCool

Thoracic Surgery Clinics (ISSN 1547-4127) is published quarterly by Elsevier Inc., 360 Park Avenue South, New York, NY 10010-1710. Months of publication are February, May, August, and November. Business and editorial offices: 1600 John F. Kennedy Boulevard, Suite 1800, Philadelphia, PA 19103-2899. Periodicals postage paid at New York, NY, and additional mailing offices. Subscription prices are $335.00 per year (US individuals), $433.00 per year (US institutions), $159.00 per year (US Students), $416.00 per year (Canadian individuals), $547.00 per year (Canadian institutions), $216.00 per year (Canadian and foreign students), $443.00 per year (foreign individuals), and $547.00 per year (foreign institutions). Foreign air speed delivery is included in all Clinics' subscription prices. All prices are subject to change without notice. **POSTMASTER:** Send address changes to Thoracic Surgery Clinics, Elsevier Health Sciences Division, Subscription Customer Service, 3251 Riverport Lane, Maryland Heights, MO 63043. **Customer Service (orders, claims, online, change of address): Telephone: 1-800-654-2452 (U.S. and Canada); 314-447-8871 (outside U.S. and Canada). Fax: 314-447-8029. Email: journalscustomerservice-usa@elsevier.com (for print support); journalsonlinesupport-usa@elsevier.com (for online support).**

Reprints. For copies of 100 or more, of articles in this publication, please contact Commercial Rights Department, Elsevier Inc., 360 Park Avenue South, New York, NY 10010-1710. Tel: (212) 633-3812; Fax: (212) 462-1935; E-mail: reprints@elsevier.com.

Thoracic Surgery Clinics is covered in *MEDLINE/PubMed (Index Medicus)* and *EMBASE/Excerpta Medica*.

Printed and bound by CPI Group (UK) Ltd, Croydon, CR0 4YY

Transferred to digital print 2012

Contributors

CONSULTING EDITOR

M. BLAIR MARSHALL, MD
Associate Professor of Surgery, Georgetown
University School of Medicine; Chief, Division
of Thoracic Surgery, Department of Surgery,
Georgetown University Medical Center,
Washington, DC

GUEST EDITOR

CLIFF K.C. CHOONG, MBBS, FRCS, FRACS
Associate Professor of Surgery, Department of
Surgery (MMC), Monash University; Consultant
Thoracic Surgeon, The Knox Hospital and
The Valley Hospital, Melbourne, Victoria,
Australia

AUTHORS

NAVEED ALAM, MD, FRCSC, FRACS
Consultant Thoracic Surgeon, Department
of Thoracic Surgery, St Vincent's
Hospital, Melbourne, Fitzroy, Victoria,
Australia

ALI AMINAZAD, MD, FRACP
Respiratory and Sleep Physician, Master of
Clinical Research Methods (Monash
University), Eastern Health, Box Hill Hospital,
Adjunct Lecturer, Monash University, Box Hill,
Melbourne, Victoria, Australia

STEPHEN R. BRODERICK, MD
Division of Cardiothoracic Surgery,
Department of Surgery, Washington
University School of Medicine, St Louis,
Missouri

CLIFF K.C. CHOONG, MBBS, FRCS, FRACS
Associate Professor of Surgery, Department of
Surgery (MMC), Monash University; Consultant
Thoracic Surgeon, The Knox Hospital and
The Valley Hospital, Melbourne, Victoria,
Australia

DAVID T. COOKE, MD, FACS
Assistant Professor, Head, General Thoracic
Surgery Program, Division of Cardiothoracic
Surgery, University of California Davis Medical
Center, Sacramento, California

ELIZABETH A. DAVID, MD
Assistant Professor, David Grant Medical
Center, USAF; Division of Cardiothoracic
Surgery, University of California Davis Medical
Center, Sacramento, California

NORMAN EIZENBERG, MBBS
Associate Professor of Anatomy, Department
of Anatomy and Developmental Biology;
Department of Surgery (MMC), Monash
University, Victoria, Australia

JACOB GILLEN, MD
Resident, Department of Surgery, University of
Virginia Health System, Charlottesville, Virginia

CHRISTINE LAU, MD, MBA
Associate Professor of Surgery, Division of
Thoracic and Cardiovascular Surgery,
Department of Surgery, University of Virginia
Health System, Charlottesville, Virginia

Y.C. GARY LEE, MBChB, PhD, FRACP, FRCP, FCCP
Department of Respiratory Medicine, Sir Charles Gairdner Hospital; Centre for Asthma, Allergy and Respiratory Research, School of Medicine and Pharmacology, University of Western Australia, Perth, Western Australia, Australia

M. BLAIR MARSHALL, MD
Associate Professor of Surgery, Georgetown University School of Medicine; Chief, Division of Thoracic Surgery, Department of Surgery, Georgetown University Medical Center, Washington, DC

SUDISH C. MURTHY, MD, PhD
Surgical Director of the Airway Center, Staff Surgeon, Department of Thoracic and Cardiovascular Surgery, Heart and Vascular Institute, Cleveland Clinic, Cleveland, Ohio

TAM QUINN, MBBS, BMedSci, PGDipSurgAnat
Royal Australasian College of Surgeons (RACS), East Melbourne; SET TRAINEE Surgical Registrar, Monash Medical Centre, Clayton, Victoria, Australia

SRIDHAR RATHINAM, FRCSEd(CTh)
Consultant Thoracic Surgeon, Department of Thoracic Surgery, Glenfield Hospital, University Hospitals of Leicester, Leicester, United Kingdom

THOMAS W. RICE, MD
Daniel and Karen Lee Endowed Chair in Thoracic Surgery, Department of Thoracic and Cardiovascular Surgery, Heart and Vascular Institute, Professor of Surgery, Cleveland Clinic Lerner College of Medicine, Cleveland Clinic, Cleveland, Ohio

VALERIE RUSCH, MD
Thoracic Surgery Service, Department of Surgery, Memorial Sloan-Kettering Cancer Center, New York, New York

RAJESH THOMAS, MBBS, FRACP
Department of Respiratory Medicine, Sir Charles Gairdner Hospital, Hospital Avenue Perth, Western Australia, Australia

DAVID A. WALLER, FRCS(CTh)
Consultant Thoracic Surgeon, Department of Thoracic Surgery, Glenfield Hospital, University Hospitals of Leicester, Leicester, United Kingdom

NILAY GAMZE YALCIN, BBioMedSc, MBBS
Department of Surgery (MMC), Monash University, Victoria, Australia

JANE YANAGAWA, MD
Thoracic Surgery Service, Department of Surgery, Memorial Sloan-Kettering Cancer Center, New York, New York

Contents

This article gives an overview of the causes and management of common benign pleural effusions.

Sudish C. Murthy and Thomas W. Rice

The two reasonable options for surgical management of malignant pleural effusions are tunneled pleural catheters and video-assisted thoracic surgery with talc pleurodesis. Successful palliation demands balancing the patient's wishes, performance status, and prognosis with the ability to obtain full lung expansion and control fluid production. There is no ideal procedure; surgical treatment must be individualized.

Sridhar Rathinam and David A. Waller

Trapped lung is defined by the inability of the lung to expand and fill the thoracic cavity because of a restricting "peel." This restriction may be secondary to a benign inflammatory or fibrotic cortex or to a malignant visceral pleural tumor. This condition has a significant impact on the patient's quality of life by causing dyspnea. This article discusses the role of surgery in relieving the trapped lung, including decortication in benign disease and pleurectomy in malignant disease. The surgical approaches of video-assisted thoracoscopy and thoracotomy are contrasted and the future potential for surgical trials in this condition is outlined.

Jacob Gillen and Christine Lau

The treatment of chronic recurrent pleural effusions continues to evolve with the recent emergence of tunneled indwelling pleural catheters (IPCs). Talc pleurodesis has been the standard of care for treatment of recurrent pleural effusions, but IPCs have gained more favor in recent years. IPCs offer several advantages, including a less invasive procedure, short postprocedure hospital stay, and greater patient control in the management of symptoms. Further randomized controlled studies are needed to more clearly differentiate which patients are better served by an IPC rather than traditional pleurodesis as their initial intervention.

Jane Yanagawa and Valerie Rusch

The uniquely diffuse nature of malignant pleural mesothelioma (MPM) makes it difficult to diagnose, stage, and treat. In addition, it is a relatively uncommon disease, making adequate prospective trials difficult to perform and leading to several controversies regarding the best management of MPM. Perhaps the greatest area of dispute is whether extrapleural pneumonectomy or pleurectomy/decortication is the most appropriate curative operation for patients who are physiologically candidates for both. Although median survival remains poor, important strides have been made in the treatment of MPM, mainly in the form of multimodality therapeutic regimens.

Stephen R. Broderick

Most cases of hemothorax are related to blunt or penetrating chest trauma. Criteria for surgical intervention for initial hemothorax are well defined. Appropriate management of retained hemothorax following initial trauma management is critical, and the best approach remains controversial. Spontaneous hemothorax is much less common and results from a variety of pathologic processes. This article reviews the etiology, diagnosis, and treatment of traumatic and spontaneous hemothorax in modern practice.

THORACIC SURGERY CLINICS

NOW AVAILABLE FOR YOUR iPhone and iPad

Preface

Management of Benign and Malignant Pleural Effusions

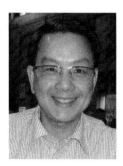

Cliff K.C. Choong, MBBS, FRCS, FRACS
Guest Editor

Pleural effusion is a common clinical problem encountered in both primary and tertiary clinical settings. There are multiple conditions that can lead to pleural effusion; hence, the investigations and tailoring an appropriate treatment are important. This issue of *Thoracic Surgery Clinics* provides a comprehensive cover on the various aspects of pleural effusion, including the anatomy of the pleural space and pleura, the pathophysiology of pleural effusion, the algorithm and decision-making in the investigations, and the management of pleural effusion. There are articles providing an update in the medical and surgical treatment of both benign and malignant pleural effusions. There are also articles focusing on the specific areas of pleural effusion, such as the treatment of malignant effusion, mesothelioma, and hemothorax. The management of patients with

trapped lung is a difficult and challenging one, and this is carefully addressed in 2 different articles looking at the role of pleurectomy and the permanent indwelling catheter. Overall, this issue of *Thoracic Surgery Clinics* provides both the basic and the advanced understanding and management of pleural effusion.

Cliff K.C. Choong, MBBS, FRCS, FRACS
Department of Surgery (MMC)
The Knox Hospital, Monash University
262 Mountain Highway
Wantirna 3152
Melbourne, Victoria, Australia

E-mail address:
cliffchoong@hotmail.com

Thorac Surg Clin 23 (2013) ix
http://dx.doi.org/10.1016/j.thorsurg.2012.11.001
1547-4127/13/$ – see front matter © 2013 Published by Elsevier Inc.

Anatomy and Pathophysiology of the Pleura and Pleural Space

Nilay Gamze Yalcin, BBioMedSc, MBBS[a],
Cliff K.C. Choong, MBBS, FRCS, FRACS[a,b,*],
Norman Eizenberg, MBBS[a,c]

KEYWORDS

- Pleura • Pleural space • Anatomy • Pathophysiology

KEY POINTS

- Pleural fluid is normally in a constant equilibrium of production and clearance.
- Pleural effusions most often arise in the setting of increased production and decreased clearance.
- The most common imaging investigations used in pleural effusions are initially chest radiographs followed by computed tomography scans.
- Ultrasound can be useful in differentiating between loculated effusions from solid masses.
- Thoracocentesis can provide more information about the underlying cause of the pleural effusion, and pleural fluid analysis can allow effusions to be classified as either transudates or exudates.
- Cytology analysis of the pleural fluid allows for the detection of malignant cells in malignant pleural effusions.

INTRODUCTION

Almost every doctor, at some stage, will have to manage a patient with pleural effusion. The complexity of pleural effusions stems from the wide range of causes that can lead to fluid buildup within the thoracic cavity. Pleural effusions are almost always secondary to a concurrent disease process occurring in the body. It is the clinicians' job to determine the nature of the underlying cause, whether that is heart failure, infection, or malignancy. Correct diagnosis will help determine the most appropriate treatment plan for the individual patient. Often, this underlying cause may not be readily apparent. This article revises the anatomy of the pleura and the physiology of pleural fluid turnover. It then explores the pathophysiology and investigations used in the workup of pleural effusions.

ANATOMY OF THE PLEURA

The pleura (derived from the Greek word for *side*) is a membrane of fibrous tissue containing a single layer of mesothelium. It aligns the interior of the thoracic cavity and is arranged into 2 layers, parietal and visceral, that are continuous at the hilum of the lung via the pulmonary ligament. The left pleural cavity does not communicate with the right side. The pulmonary ligament hangs inferiorly from the hilum of each lung as a double fold of pleura and creates an empty space that allows for the expansion of vessels in the lung hilum as the diaphragm descends with inspiration.

The pleural space contains a small amount of fluid between its outer parietal and inner visceral layers to maintain apposition during respiration.[1] This pleural fluid secreted and reabsorbed from the potential space between the visceral and

---

[a] Department of Surgery (MMC), Monash University, Clayton Road, Victoria 3800, Australia; [b] The Knox Hospital and The Valley Hospital, 262 Mountain Highway, Wantirna 3152, Melbourne, Victoria, Australia; [c] Department of Anatomy and Developmental Biology, Monash University, Wellington Road, Victoria 3800, Australia
* Corresponding author. The Knox Hospital and The Valley Hospital, 262 Mountain Highway, Wantirna 3152, Melbourne, Victoria, Australia.
E-mail address: cliffchoong@hotmail.com

Thorac Surg Clin 23 (2013) 1–10
http://dx.doi.org/10.1016/j.thorsurg.2012.10.008
1547-4127/13/$ – see front matter © 2013 Published by Elsevier Inc.

parietal layers assists in creating a negative intra-thoracic pressure, which preserves lung inflation during inspiration. However, the entry of air or the accumulation of fluid may lead to mechanical dysfunction of breathing, as discussed later.

The visceral pleura is adherent to the lung parenchyma from the hila outward and lines the transverse and oblique fissures. The parietal pleura lines the interior surface of the thoracic wall and is separated from it by the underlying endothoracic fascia. This thin extrapleural layer of connective tissue provides a surgical plane for the separation of the parietal pleura from the thoracic wall. The endothoracic fascia also separates the diaphragm from the parietal pleura. The parietal pleura, however, is strongly adherent to the fibrous pericardium and diaphragm and has no accessible surgical plane at these sites.[2]

SURFACE MARKINGS OF THE PLEURA

The outline of the parietal pleura can be traced along the thoracic wall by using the even-numbered ribs[2–7] as external landmarks to visualize the distribution (**Fig. 1**). The parietal pleura extends 2.5 cm above the medial third of the clavicle. The line of pleural reflection on both right and left sides then project down inferomedially from behind the sternoclavicular joint to meet at the sternal angle located at the level of the second costal cartilage. The parietal pleura then continues vertically down to the fourth costal cartilage. From here, the left side deviates laterally toward the border of the sternum. It continues half way to the apex of the heart, whereas

the direction of the right side remains unchanged. The parietal pleura on both sides turns laterally after crossing the sixth rib. The parietal pleura crosses the eighth rib at the midclavicular line and crosses the tenth rib at the midaxillary line. At the level of the twelfth rib, the parietal pleura is located at the lateral border of erector spinae. From here, it passes horizontally toward the twelfth thoracic vertebra, resulting in the pleura being located behind the upper pole of the kidney, particularly on the left, which is a clinically significant consideration in the scenario of wounds or incisions at this site. The lungs, however, do not reach as far down as the parietal pleurae, which creates the costodiaphragmatic recess on each side.[1]

Although the pleura is protected by the bony thoracic cavity, there are 3 sites where it extends beyond the rib cage and is particularly vulnerable to penetrating injury, including surgery whereby infection and/or air may be introduced into the pleural space, as shown in **Fig. 2**.[1]

1. Above the medial end of the first rib onto the root of the neck bilaterally as cervical pleura (may also puncture lung apex)
2. Below the costo-xiphisternal angle on the right side
3. Below the costovertebral angle on bilaterally

The visceral pleura receives an autonomic nerve supply, which is insensitive to most stimuli. In contrast, the innervation of the parietal pleura is somatic, thus, highly sensitive. The parietal pleura can be divided into 4 parts (costal, mediastinal, cervical, and diaphragmatic) via the *lines of pleural reflection*, which occur when the costal pleura becomes

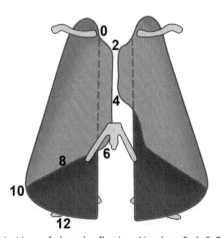

Fig. 1. Lines of pleural reflection. Numbers 2, 4, 6, 8, 10 and 12 correspond to the overlying costal cartilage or rib, 0 represents the clavicle. (*From* Eizenberg N, Briggs C, Barker P, et al. Anatomedia 'a new approach to medical education developments in anatomy': thorax (regions). McGraw-Hill; 2012. Available at: www.anatomedia.com. Accessed October 10, 2012; with permission.)

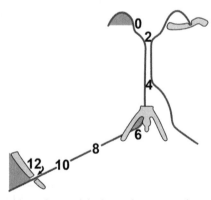

Fig. 2. Pleura beyond the bony thorax. Numbers 2, 4, 6, 8, 10 and 12 correspond to the overlying costal cartilage or rib, 0 represents the clavicle. (*From* Eizenberg N, Briggs C, Barker P, et al. Anatomedia 'a new approach to medical education developments in anatomy': thorax (regions). McGraw-Hill; 2012. Available at: www.anatomedia.com. Accessed October 10, 2012; with permission.)

of the pleural reflections possesses an individual innervation and referred pain profile. The cervical pleura rises to the neck of the first rib. Like the costal pleura, the innervation is provided by the thoracic spinal nerves. Although irritation of the costal pleura will refer pain to the skin overlying the thorax, the cervical pleura is predominantly supplied by the first thoracic spinal nerve, thus, it may refer pain to the inner aspect of the upper limb when irritated.

As the phrenic nerve (C3, 4, 5) runs down beside the fibrous pericardium toward the diaphragm, it provides somatic sensation for both the mediastinal as well as the central part of the diaphragmatic pleura and classically refers pain to the ipsilateral shoulder tip via the C4 dermatome. In contrast, the peripheral areas of the diaphragmatic pleura receive their nerve supply from the lower 6 thoracic spinal nerves and may refer pain to the anterior abdominal wall.[1]

BLOOD SUPPLY AND LYMPHATICS

Similar to its innervation, the vascular system of the parietal pleura is also derived from somatic sources. The arterial supply is provided through the intercostal, internal thoracic, and musculophrenic arteries. The anterior intercostal arteries arise from both the internal thoracic artery and its terminating branch, the musculophrenic artery. The posterior intercostal arteries generally arise off the descending aorta with the exception of the first two, which branch off from the subclavian artery. The venous drainage of parietal pleura occurs through intercostal veins. The second to eleventh anterior intercostal veins drain into the internal thoracic veins, the supreme intercostal vein drains into the brachiocephalic vein, and the posterior intercostal veins drain into the azygos venous system.

The lymphatics of the parietal pleura drain into the intercostal, parasternal, diaphragmatic, and posterior mediastinal group of nodes.

The visceral pleura, however, has its arterial supply and venous drainage from the bronchial vessels, similar to the lung parenchyma to which it is adherent. The lymphatics drain toward the nodes of the lungs. The lungs of city dwellers often show hexagonal carbon deposits, which represent the subpleural lymphatic system in which inhaled carbon has become trapped (**Fig. 3**).[8]

ANATOMIC VARIATIONS

Common variations may impact on the anatomy of the pleura, such as the presence of accessory lung lobes, azygos venous system variations, and the presence of a lateral costal artery.

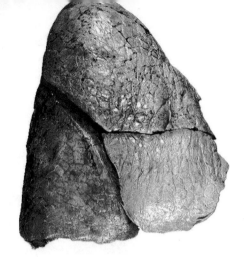

Fig. 3. Carbon deposits in subpleural lymphatics. (*From* Eizenberg N, Briggs C, Barker P, et al. Anatomedia 'a new approach to medical education developments in anatomy': thorax (systems). McGraw-Hill; 2012. Available at: www.anatomedia.com. Accessed October 10, 2012; with permission.)

The azygos venous system, a highly variable anatomic structure, comprises the azygos, hemiazygos, and accessory hemiazygos veins. In a rare anatomic variation, the arch of the azygos vein may be displaced laterally, which creates a pleural septum. This septum separates the upper right lobe and creates what is known as the azygos lobe. Other accessory lobes occur because of the developmental anomalies in the lung fissures. Common accessory lobes include posterior accessory, inferior accessory, and the middle lobe of left lung.[3] In the case of accessory lung lobes, the visceral pleura continues to align the surfaces and fissures created by the lobe. The parietal pleura is normally not affected in these cases.

Additionally, in about 25% of cases, a lateral costal artery runs down the internal aspect of the anterior chest wall (**Fig. 4**). The lateral costal artery is a branch of the internal thoracic artery arising from it behind the first costal cartilage and terminating in the fourth, fifth, or sixth intercostal space by anastomosing with a posterior intercostal artery.[1]

PHYSIOLOGY OF PLEURAL FLUID

Pleural fluid is in a constant equilibrium of production and absorption within the pleural space. It is estimated that the fluid is produced, on average, at 0.01 mL/kg/h and cleared at the same rate, keeping its volume in the pleural space constant.[9] It follows that, over a 24-hour period, the average 60-kg person will have 14.4 mL of pleural fluid turnover.

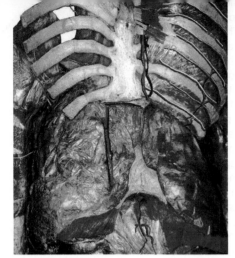

Fig. 4. Anterior thoracic wall reflected upwards with left internal thoracic and left lateral costal vessels shown on its internal aspect (arteries: red; veins: blue; lymph nodes: orange; nerves: yellow). Right internal thoracic and right lateral costal vessels shown on external aspect of parietal pleura. (*From* Eizenberg N, Briggs C, Barker P, et al. Anatomedia 'a new approach to medical education developments in anatomy': thorax (dissection). McGraw-Hill; 2012. Available at: www.anatomedia.com. Accessed October 10, 2012; with permission.)

Within the normal physiologic process, the parietal pleura seems to have a more crucial role in pleural fluid homeostasis.[4] Its vessels are closer to the pleural space (10–12 μm) compared with that of the visceral pleura (20–50 μm), and the filtration pressures are likely to be higher. Additionally, the parietal pleura is consistent across species compared with the highly variable visceral pleura. The parietal pleura also seems to be responsible for the clearance of pleural fluid because it contains multiple lymphatic stomata, 1 to 6 μm in diameter which open directly into the pleural space.[5,10] These stomata are exclusively present on the parietal pleura.[4] The hypothesis remains that most of the pleural filtrate is reabsorbed by these parietal lymphatics supported by the fact that studies show a bulk clearance of the fluid rather than a diffusional process. A portion is reabsorbed by the venules and the remainder stays in the pleural space. Additionally, there is a large reserve for reabsorption in response to increased production, which can increase reabsorption rates from 0.01 mL/kg/hr to as high as 0.28 mL/kg/hr.[5]

PATHOPHYSIOLOGY OF PLEURAL FLUID ACCUMULATION

Pleural effusions occur when there is too much production or too little absorption of the fluid in the pleural space, usually a combination ﹏ Fluid may also come from the peritoneum v﹏ in the diaphragm.[11]

The Starling equation can be applied her﹏ termine the forces that effect pleural fluid b﹏

$$Flow = k \times ([Pmv - Ppmv] - s [\pi mv - $$

Where

- *k* is the liquid conductance of the mi﹏ cular barrier
- *Pmv* is the hydrostatic pressure ﹏ microvascular compartment
- *Ppmv* is the hydrostatic pressure in t﹏ microvascular compartment
- *s* is the reflection coefficient for total﹏ (range 0–1)
- *πmv* is protein osmotic pressure﹏ microvascular compartment
- *πpmv* is protein osmotic pressure﹏ peri-microvascular compartment

Therefore, effusions may be caused by an i﹏ in permeability (increased k or decreased s)﹏ to an exudative pleural effusion.

Alternatively, there may be a widening﹏ hydrostatic versus oncotic pressures lea﹏ a transudative pleural effusion. Transudati﹏ sions may be caused by

- Systemic microvascular pressure in﹏
- Decreased pleural pressure
- Lowered systemic protein concentr﹏
- Increased pleural fluid protein (not c﹏ significant)

History and Examination

Pleural effusions may cause dyspnea, ﹏ pain, or, alternatively, be asymptomatic. A ﹏ history needs to include comorbidities th﹏ lead to pleural effusions; potential occu﹏ exposures, such as asbestos; and a deta﹏ of medications and other drugs. Often du﹏ clinical examination, the side of the che﹏ the effusion will have reduced or absent﹏ sounds with evidence of bronchial brea﹏ the compressed lung tissue directly overl﹏ fluid collection. Percussion of the fluid w﹏ stony dullness. Additionally, there may be a﹏ tion on chest expansion on the affect﹏ alongside reduced vocal resonance.

When a pleural effusion is suspected, im﹏ the best initial modality to confirm the clinic﹏ cion. The chest radiograph is the most c﹏ modality, followed by computed tomogra﹏ or ultrasound. Thoracocentesis may be u﹏ further define the cause of the effusion.

DIAGNOSIS
Imaging

Chest radiographs
As free-moving fluid, pleural effusions initially collect at the subpulmonic area between the inferior surface of the lower lobes and the diaphragmatic leaflets. Up to 75 mL can collect in this area before it spills over into the costophrenic sulcus. Once this spillover occurs, the fluid is observable from a plain upright chest radiograph creating a meniscoid arc where the fluid makes contact with the parietal pleura. As little as 75 mL can obscure the posterior costophrenic sulcus, whereas 175 mL is necessarily for the lateral costophrenic sulcus.[12] Once the diaphragm becomes obscured, the pleural fluid has reached 500 mL; if it is as high as the anterior aspect of the fourth rib, the fluid volume has reached 1000 mL.

Volumes as little as 5 mL may be detected on a decubitus radiograph, with 10 mL being easily seen.[7] On the decubitus view, the amount of effusion can be classified as small (<1.5 cm), moderate (1.5–4.5 cm), or large (>4.5 cm).[13]

For patients who have a supine chest radiograph, pleural effusions become visible once the volume reaches 175 mL.[14] If mobile, the effusion may track along the posterior thorax creating a deceptively similar appearance to preexisting lung disease, pneumonia, or atelectasis in critically ill patients for whom supine imaging is most often ordered.[13]

Subpulmonic effusions Subpulmonic effusions, best seen on a lateral view, cause an increase in the lung base, which may give the appearance of a raised diaphragmatic leaflet.[15] The radiographic appearance has been likened to the Rock of Gibraltar because the natural curvature of the hemidiaphragm seems to be displaced laterally, creating a sharp dip as it reaches the costophrenic angle. An increased separation (>2 cm) on the left side between the lower aspect of the lung and the stomach bubble raises suspicion for this type of effusion, particularly if seen in the frontal and lateral views.

Loculated pleural effusions Loculated pleural effusions occur in the presence of adhesions and may be mistaken for a mass. They occur most commonly in the setting of pyothorax, hemothorax, chylothorax and tuberculous pleuritis and possess the following typical features[12]:

- Homogenous appearance
- Drooping on upright imaging caused by its fluid nature

- Obtuse angles at the interface between the apparent mass and chest wall
- Distinct surface: smooth if visualized in tangent, poor if visualized en face, and partially visualized in oblique (incomplete border sign)

CT
Chest CT, although not the first line, is useful in determining the size and location of the pleural effusion. Its multiple other uses include identifying the following[16–18]:

- Pleural thickness or masses
- Empyema
- Small pneumothorax in supine patients
- Lung masses or parenchymal processes
- Mass location and composition
- Pleural effusion cause
- Guidance for thoracocentesis and drain insertion for loculated pleural collection
- Peripheral bronchopleural fistulae
- Diaphragmatic defects in hepatic hydrothorax

Ultrasound
Ultrasound has a place in guiding a thoracocentesis as well as differentiating loculated effusions from solid masses.[19]

Thoracocentesis

Once an effusion is established on imaging, in selected patients, a thoracocentesis is performed depending on the clinical condition of the patients and physician choice to elucidate the nature and cause of the effusion. A study performed by Collins and colleagues[20] showed that thoracocentesis provided a definitive diagnosis in 18% of cases and confirmed the pretest clinical impression in another 56%. Overall, it allowed for better clinical decision making in up to 90% of cases. The diagnoses, which can be established using a thoracocentesis, are shown in the **Table 1**.[21,22]

Pleural fluid analysis
Gross appearance The observations, which may be helpful in diagnosis, are shown in **Table 2**.[21]

Transudate or exudate
The characterization of the pleural effusion as a transudate or an exudate can be helpful in determining the cause. Traditionally, Light's criteria have been used to establish the nature of the fluid.

Exudates meet at least one of Light's criterion, whereas transudates meet none[23]:

1. Pleural fluid protein to serum protein ratio greater than 0.5

Table 1
Diagnosis that can be established via thoracocentesis with corresponding pleural fluid test

Condition	Diagnostic Analysis of Pleural Fluid Sample
Empyema	Distinct appearance (pus, putrid odor) Positive culture
Malignancy	Positive cytology for malignant cells
Hemothorax	Blood or fluid with hematocrit (pleural fluid-to-blood ratio >0.5)
Chylothorax	Chyle fluid with triglycerides Lipoprotein electrophoresis
Lupus pleuritis	Pleural fluid serum ANA >1.0 LE cells
Tuberculous pleurisy	Positive AFB stain Positive culture
Fungal pleurisy	Positive KOH stain Positive culture
Esophageal rupture	High salivary amylase Pleural fluid acidosis (often as low as 6.00)
Urinothorax	Creatinine (pleural fluid/serum >1.0)
Peritoneal dialysis	Protein (<1 g/dL) Glucose (300–400 mg/dL)

Abbreviations: AFB, Acid-fast bacillus; ANA, antinuclear antibody; KOH, potassium hydroxide; LE, lupus erythematosus.

2. Pleural fluid LDH to serum LDH ratio greater than 0.6
3. Pleural fluid LDH greater than two-thirds of the upper limit of normal for serum

The aforementioned criteria misdiagnoses 20% of transudates as exudative. If the clinical suspicion is that the fluid is a transudate, the albumin levels between the serum and the pleural fluid

Table 2
Causes of pleural effusion with corresponding color, character, and odor profiles

	Potential Diagnosis
Color of Fluid	
Pale yellow (straw)	Transudate in general, occasionally some clear exudative fluid
Red (bloody)	Hemothorax, bloody malignant effusion, asbestos-related pleural effusion, postcardiac injury syndrome, or pulmonary infarction in absence of trauma
White (milky)	Chylous fluid or cholesterol effusion
Brown	Long-standing bloody effusion, rupture of amoebic liver abscess
Black	Fungal, such as *Aspergillus*
Yellow-green	Rheumatoid pleurisy
Dark green	Biliary fluid (Biliothorax)
Character of Fluid	
Thick yellow	Pus (empyema)
Viscous	Malignant pleural effusion (metastatic malignancy or mesothelioma)
Debris	Rheumatoid pleurisy
Turbid	Infective or inflammatory exudate or lipid effusion
Anchovy paste	Amoebic liver abscess
Odor of Fluid	
Putrid	Anaerobic empyema
Ammonia	Urinothorax

can be compared. For example, diuresis in heart failure can cause an increase in protein levels putting it in the exudative range; but a serum–pleural fluid albumin gradient more than 1.2 g/dL can be used to categorize the effusion as a transudate.[24,25] An additional supporting factor for a transudative pleural effusion in the setting of heart failure is high N-terminal pro–brain natriuretic peptide (NT-proBNP).[26]

Protein Under normal physiologic conditions, the pleural fluid has a protein content of 0.25 mL/kg. Transudates have a protein level less than 3.0 g/dL, with some exceptions (eg, diuresis in heart failure as discussed earlier).[24]

In comparison, exudates have high protein concentrations. For example, protein levels of 7.0 to 8.0 g/dL raise the suspicion of Walderström macroglobulinemia and multiple myeloma, whereas tuberculous effusions most commonly show a protein concentration of more than 4.0 g/dL.[23,27,28]

Lactate dehydrogenase The upper limit of normal for serum lactate dehydrogenase (LDH) is 200 IU/L. If the pleural fluid LDH is significantly elevated (>1000 IU/L), the potential culprits include[29–31]

- Rheumatoid pleurisy
- Empyema
- Pleural paragonimiasis
- Malignancy

Cholesterol The most common source of cholesterol in the pleural fluid is from degenerating cells or from vascular sources as a consequence of increased permeability. This phenomenon commonly occurs in long-standing pleural disease. Cholesterol effusions (also known as chyliform effusions or pseudochylothorax) classically display pleural cholesterol levels greater than 200 mg/dL and a cholesterol-to-triglyceride ratio greater than 1.[32]

Triglycerides The presence of more than 110 mg/dL of triglycerides in the pleural fluid indicates a chylothorax. When the triglyceride level is less than 50 mg/dL, a chylothorax can safely be ruled out; but a lipoprotein analysis is required if the levels lie between these two figures.[33]

Glucose Transudates and most exudates have a similar glucose level to that of serum. However, some exceptions apply. In the setting of exudative effusions, a low glucose level (<60 mg/dL) or pleural fluid–to–serum glucose ratio greater than 0.5 makes the following diagnosis most likely[34]:

- Lupus pleuritis
- Rheumatoid pleurisy
- Complicated parapneumonic effusion/empyema

- Esophageal rupture
- Malignant effusion
- Tuberculous pleurisy

pH The pleural fluid pH is best measured in a blood gas machine.[35] The causes of a low pleural fluid pH (less than 7.30) in the setting of a normal blood pH are the same differentials as those of low glucose, listed earlier.[36]

Amylase This test is not routine because it has a little role in determining benign from malignant effusions but may be requested in certain clinical situations. Raised amylase may be a result of[37]

- Esophageal rupture
- Chronic pancreatic pleural effusion
- Acute pancreatitis
- Malignancy
- Rarely, pneumonia, hydronephrosis, or cirrhosis[38]

Adenosine deaminase When the initial cytology, smear, and culture of an exudative effusion are negative, the adenosine deaminase (ADA) levels may be used to differentiate malignancy from tuberculous pleurisy. The ADA levels in the setting of tuberculous pleurisy are usually more than 35 to 50 U/L.[39] ADA levels must be evaluated with the patient's history and clinical presentation in mind because false positives and negatives can occur.

NT pro-BNP Heart failure and concurrent pleural effusion cause an elevation in the NT pro-BNP levels.[40] However, there is a high correlation between serum and pleural fluid NT pro-BNP levels; thus, there has been no established benefit to measuring pleural fluid NT pro-BNP values over serum values.[26]

Tumor markers There is currently no pleural fluid tumor marker that is accurate enough to be used routinely in pleural fluid analysis. Individual markers that may be assessed include

- Carbohydrate antigen (CA) 15–3
- CA 19–9
- Carcinoembryonic antigen
- CA 125
- Cytokeratin fragment 21–1
- Mesothelin and mesothelin-related peptides

Nucleated cells The nucleated cell count is not usually diagnostic but may give certain clues:

- Only complicated parapneumonic effusions (including empyema) exhibit nucleated cell counts more than 50 000/μL

- Bacterial pneumonia, lupus pleuritis, and acute pancreatitis are exudates that typically exhibit nucleated cell counts greater than 10 000/μL
- Chronic exudate, often show nucleated cell counts less than 5000/μL (eg, malignancy, tuberculous pleurisy)[37]

Lymphocytosis Pleural fluid lymphocytosis, especially when lymphocytes compose 85% to 95% of nucleated cells, may be caused by the following[21,37,41]:

- Chronic rheumatoid pleurisy
- Tuberculous pleurisy
- Sarcoidosis
- Chylothorax
- Lymphoma

Malignant pleural effusions exhibit lymphocytosis in half of the cases, but the magnitude of lymphocytosis is between 50% and 70% in these cases.[41]

Eosinophilia Eosinophilia of pleural fluid is characteristically defined as the presence of greater than 10% of total nucleated cells. Usually, eosinophilia of pleural fluid is caused by the presence of air or blood as a result of benign disease.[42] Differentials for pleural fluid eosinophilia include the following:

- Pneumothorax
- Pulmonary infarction
- Hemothorax
- Malignancy (carcinoma, lymphoma)
- Benign asbestos pleural effusion
- Drugs
- Parasitic disease
- Fungal infection (coccidioidomycosis, cryptococcosis, histoplasmosis)
- Catamenial pneumothorax with pleural effusion

Mesothelial cells A small number of mesothelial cells are normally found in pleural fluid. In transudative effusions, the mesothelial cell count is high, whereas the presence of mesothelial cells is rather varied with exudative effusions. Of clinical relevance, mesothelial cell count greater than 5% in an exudative effusion makes tuberculosis an unlikely diagnosis.[43]

SPECIFIC TYPES OF PLEURAL EFFUSIONS
Transudates

Left ventricular failure is the most common cause of transudative pleural effusions, with 90% being bilateral.[12] Constrictive pericarditis, cirrhosis, and renal failure are among other causes of transudative effusions. In the setting of cirrhosis, a hepatic

hydrothorax is diagnosed if there is no identifiable pulmonary, pleural, or cardiac disease to account for the fluid buildup. Hepatic hydrothorax is commonly located on the right side.

Exudates

Commonly seen exudative pleural effusions are caused by empyema, malignancy, chylothorax, and hemothorax. These conditions are discussed later.

Empyema

Empyema is most commonly a complication following pulmonary infections, occurring typically in the postpneumonic or parapneumonic period. Other causes include surgical procedures and trauma. Commonly, they are caused by anaerobes or an anaerobe-aerobe combination.

Empyema can be classified in 3 stages:

1. Exudative stage: pleural membrane swelling
2. Fibrinopurulent stage: adhesions formation
3. Organizing stage: collagen deposition, development of a thick pleural peel

The significance of the stages is that it can help determine the best treatment modality. Stage 1 is drainable, but stage 2 would require thoracic surgical drainage and stage 3 may need decortication. On imaging, staging 2 and 3 show pleural thickening greater than 3 to 5 mm and demonstrates the split pleura sign on CT.[17]

Additionally, there may be a gas-fluid level associated with the empyema, which could signify a bronchopulmonary fistula (BPF). Usually peripheral BPF are complications of necrotizing pneumonia, whereas centrally located BPF are caused by trauma or surgical procedures and they can sometimes be confirmed on bronchoscopy.[18]

Malignant pleural effusions

Malignancy represents the second most common cause of exudative pleural effusions.[44,45] Cancer of the lung, breast, ovary, or lymphoma make up 80% of the primary malignancies. Mechanisms leading to an effusion include

- Obstruction of the lymphatic system
- Increase in the permeability of capillaries and pleural membranes
- Bronchial obstruction causing atelectasis (leading to fluid accumulation around the affected region caused by decreased local pressure)

Malignant effusions, on CT, exhibit irregular, nodular, or thickened pleura. They may even opacify a hemithorax or become loculated.

A positive pleural biopsy and/or pleural fluid cytology result indicates a malignant effusion. In the cases when the pleural fluid cytology and pleural biopsy are negative, the effusion is termed a paramalignant pleural effusion.

Hemothorax

Hemothorax is defined as bloodstained pleural effusion containing a hematocrit level that is greater than half of the value in the peripheral blood.[12] Leading causes include anticoagulants, pulmonary emboli, metastatic processes, and trauma.

Chylothorax

Lymphoma and lung cancer make up 54% of the cases of chylothorax, with another 10% caused by surgical trauma.[46] Other causes include lymphangioleiomyomatosis, filariasis, idiopathic chylothorax, and congenital anomalies of the thoracic duct.

In the setting of trauma, a right-sided chylothorax indicates damage to the lower third of the thoracic duct and the left-sided chylothorax indicates damage to the upper two-thirds of the thoracic duct because the thoracic duct crosses the from right to left as it ascends.

Additional Testing

Despite the investigations discussed earlier, the cause of a pleural effusion is not determined in up to 25% of cases. In these cases, it is crucial to go back to the patients' history and concentrate on drugs, occupational exposures, and any comorbidities that may predispose to pleural effusions. It is important to specifically elicit the patients' pulmonary embolus risk and potential tuberculosis exposure. The pleural fluid may be sent off for a second analysis. If not done, a CT with pleural phase contrast enhancement may provide further imaging details. It may show irregularities or thickening of the pleura consistent with a malignant or inflammatory process. It can also show an underlying pathologic condition that may have precipitated the effusion. Additionally, it will assist in determining the best pleural biopsy site. Pleural biopsy may also be performed with ultrasound guidance or thoracoscopy.

SUMMARY

Pleural fluid is normally in a constant equilibrium of production and clearance. Pleural effusions most often arise in the setting of increased production and decreased clearance. The most common imaging investigations used in pleural effusions are chest radiographs and CT scans. Ultrasound can be useful in differentiating loculated effusions from solid masses. Thoracocentesis can provide more detail about the underlying cause of the pleural effusion. Pleural fluid analysis can allow effusions to be classified as either transudates or exudates.

REFERENCES

1. Eizenberg N, Briggs C, Barker P, et al. Anatomedia 'a new approach to medical education developments in anatomy': thorax (regions). McGraw-Hill; 2012. Available at: www.anatomedia.com. Accessed October 10, 2012.
2. Shields TW. Anatomy of the pleura. In: Shields TW, Locicero J, Ponn RB, et al, editors. General thoracic surgery, vol. 1, 6th edition. Philadelphia: Lippincott Williams & Wilkins; 2005. p. 786.
3. Shields TW. Surgical anatomy of the lung. In: Shields TW, Locicero J, Ponn RB, et al, editors. General thoracic surgery, vol. 1, 6th edition. Philadelphia: Lippincott Williams & Wilkins; 2005. p. 59–60.
4. Staub NC, Wiener-Kronish JP, Albertine KH. Transport through the pleura: physiology of normal liquid and solute exchange in the pleural space. In: Chretien J, Bignon J, Hirsch A, editors. The pleura in health and disease. New York: Marcel Dekker; 1985. p. 169–93.
5. Broaddus VC, Weiner-Kronish JP, Berthiaume Y, et al. Removal of pleural liquid and protein by lymphatics in awake sheep. J Appl Physiol 1988;64:384.
6. Starling EH. On the absorption of fluids from the connective tissue spaces. J Physiol 1896;19:312.
7. Moskowitz H, Platt RT, Schachar R, et al. Roentgen visualization of minute pleural effusion. An experimental study to determine the minimum amount of pleural fluid visible on a radiograph. Radiology 1973;109:33.
8. Eizenberg N, Briggs C, Barker P, et al. Anatomedia: 'a new approach to medical education developments in anatomy': thorax (systems). McGraw-Hill; 2012. Available at: www.anatomedia.com. Accessed October 10, 2012.
9. Weiner-Kronish JP, Albertine KH, Licko V, et al. Protein egress and entry rates in pleural fluid and plasma in sheep. J Appl Physiol 1984;56:459.
10. Albertine KH, Wiener-Kronish JP, Staub NC. The structure of the parietal pleura and its relationship to pleural liquid dynamics in sheep. Anat Rec 1984;208:401.
11. Lieberman FL, Hidemura R, Peters RL, et al. Pathogenesis and treatment of hydrothorax complicating cirrhosis with ascites. Ann Intern Med 1966;64:341.
12. Stark P. The pleura. In: Taveras JM, Ferrucci JT, editors. Radiology. Diagnosis imaging, intervention. Philadelphia: Lippincott; 2000. p. 1–29.
13. Ruskin JA, Gurney JW, Thorsen MK, et al. Detection of pleural effusions on supine chest radiographs. AJR Am J Roentgenol 1987;148:681.

14. Woodring JH. Recognition of pleural effusion on supine radiographs: how much fluid is required? AJR Am J Roentgenol 1984;142:59–64.

15. Eisenberg RL, Johnson NM. Comprehensive Radiographic Pathology. 5th edition. Missouri: Elsevier; 2012. p. 78.

16. Evans AL, Gleeson FV. Radiology in pleural disease: state of the art. Respirology 2004;9:300.

17. Stark DD, Federle MP, Goodman PC, et al. Differentiating lung abscess and empyema: radiography and computed tomography. AJR Am J Roentgenol 1983;141:163.

18. Westcott JL, Volpe JP. Peripheral bronchopleural fistula: CT evaluation in 20 patients with pneumonia, empyema, or postoperative air leak. Radiology 1995;196:175.

19. Moore CL, Copel JA. Point-of-care ultrasonography. N Engl J Med 2011;364:749.

20. Collins TR, Sahn SA. Thoracocentesis. Clinical value, complications, technical problems, and patient experience. Chest 1987;91:817.

21. Sahn SA. The diagnostic value of pleural fluid analysis. Semin Respir Crit Care Med 1995;16:269.

22. Ali HA, Lippmann M, Mundathaje U, et al. Spontaneous hemothorax: a comprehensive review. Chest 2008;134:1056.

23. Light RW, Macgregor MI, Luchsinger PC, et al. Pleural effusions: the diagnostic separation of transudates and exudates. Ann Intern Med 1972;77:507.

24. Romero-Candeira S, Fernández C, Martín C, et al. Influence of diuretics on the concentration of proteins and other components of pleural transudates in patients with heart failure. Am J Med 2001;110:681.

25. Roth BJ, O'Meara TF, Cragun WH. The serum-effusion albumin gradient in the evaluation of pleural effusions. Chest 1990;98:546.

26. Porcel JM. Utilization of B-type natriuretic peptide and NT-proBNP in the diagnosis of pleural effusions due to heart failure. Curr Opin Pulm Med 2011;17:215.

27. Winterbauer RH, Riggins RC, Griesman FA, et al. Pleuropulmonary manifestations of Waldenstrom's macroglobulinemia. Chest 1974;66:368.

28. Rodríguez JN, Pereira A, Martínez JC, et al. Pleural effusion in multiple myeloma. Chest 1994;105:622.

29. Light RW, Girard WM, Jenkinson SG, et al. Parapneumonic effusions. Am J Med 1980;69:507.

30. Pettersson T, Klockars M, Hellström PE. Chemical and immunological features of pleural effusions: comparison between rheumatoid arthritis and other diseases. Thorax 1982;37:354.

31. Johnson JR, Falk A, Iber C, et al. Paragonimiasis in the United States. A report of nine cases in Hmong immigrants. Chest 1982;82:168.

32. Huggins JT. Chylothorax and cholesterol pleural effusion. Semin Respir Crit Care Med 2010;31:743.

33. Staats BA, Ellefson RD, Budahn LL, et al. The lipoprotein profile of chylous and nonchylous pleural effusions. Mayo Clin Proc 1980;55:700.

34. Sahn SA. Pathogenesis and clinical features of diseases associated with a low pleural fluid glucose. In: Chretien J, Bignon J, Hirsch A, editors. The pleura in health and disease. New York: Marcel Dekker; 1985. p. 267–85.

35. Cheng DS, Rodriguez RM, Rogers J, et al. Comparison of pleural fluid pH values obtained using blood gas machine, pH meter, and pH indicator strip. Chest 1998;114:1368.

36. Sahn SA. Pleural fluid pH in the normal state and in diseases affecting the pleural space. In: Chretien J, Bignon J, Hirsch A, editors. The pleura in health and disease. New York: Marcel Dekker; 1985. p. 253.

37. Sahn SA. State of the art. The pleura. Am Rev Respir Dis 1988;138:184.

38. Joseph J, Viney S, Beck P, et al. A prospective study of amylase-rich pleural effusions with special reference to amylase isoenzyme analysis. Chest 1992; 102:1455.

39. Riantawan P, Chaowalit P, Wongsangiem M, et al. Diagnostic value of pleural fluid adenosine deaminase in tuberculous pleuritis with reference to HIV coinfection and a Bayesian analysis. Chest 1999;116:97.

40. Janda S, Swiston J. Diagnostic accuracy of pleural fluid NT-pro-BNP for pleural effusions of cardiac origin: a systematic review and meta-analysis. BMC Pulm Med 2010;10:58.

41. Yam LT. Diagnostic significance of lymphocytes in pleural effusions. Ann Intern Med 1967;66:972.

42. Adelman M, Albelda SM, Gottlieb J, et al. Diagnostic utility of pleural fluid eosinophilia. Am J Med 1984; 77:915.

43. Light RW, Erozan YS, Ball WC Jr. Cells in pleural fluid. Their value in differential diagnosis. Arch Intern Med 1973;132:854.

44. Chernow B, Sahn SA. Carcinomatous involvement of the pleura: an analysis of 96 patients. Am J Med 1977;63:695.

45. Fentiman IS, Millis R, Sexton S, et al. Pleural effusion in breast cancer: a review of 105 cases. Cancer 1981;47:2087.

46. Roy PH, Carr DT, Payne WS. The problem of chylothorax. Mayo Clin Proc 1967;42:457.

Decision Making and Algorithm for the Management of Pleural Effusions

Tam Quinn, MBBS, BMedSci, PGDipSurgAnat[a,b],
Naveed Alam, MD, FRCSC, FRACS[c], Ali Aminazad, MD, FRACP[d],
M. Blair Marshall, MD[e],
Cliff K.C. Choong, MBBS, FRCS, FRACS[f,g],*

KEYWORDS

- Pleural effusion • Management • Causes • Algorithm

KEY POINTS

- Multiple causes for pleural effusion ranging from cardiovascular disease to infection to neoplasm.
- History and examination can elicit cause. Radiological investigations are a useful adjunct to diagnosis.
- Management varies depending on diagnosis, from treatment of underlying cause to symptomatic treatment.

INTRODUCTION

The pleural space, between the visceral and parietal pleura, usually contains between 10 to 25 mL of fluid.[1] This fluid is a filtrate created in the pleural capillaries and lymphatics and is largely reabsorbed via the lymphatics of the parietal pleura.[2] In disease states, more than 3 L of fluid can accumulate within the pleural cavity. Pleural diseases are common, and more than 3000 per 1 million population develop a pleural effusion each year. Considering that there are 60 different causes of pleural effusions, establishing the diagnosis and subsequent management can be challenging.[3] Left ventricular failure is the most common cause,[1,2] and other causes are categorized and listed later.

Part I: Pathogenesis and Causes of Pleural Effusions

Pathogenesis

The pathogenesis of pleural effusions can largely be classified as excess pleural fluid formation or decreased fluid reabsorption. In greater detail, the mechanisms of the development of pleural effusions can be caused by the following[2,4]:

- Increased pulmonary capillary pressure (eg, heart failure)
- Increased pulmonary capillary permeability (eg, pneumonia)
- Decreased intrapleural pressure (eg, atelectasis)
- Decreased plasma oncotic pressure (eg, hypoalbuminemia)

[a] Royal Australasian College of Surgeons (RACS), College of Surgeons' Gardens, 250-290 Spring Street, East Melbourne, VIC 3002, Australia; [b] Department of Cardiothoracic Surgery, Monash Medical Centre, 246 Clayton Road, Clayton 3002, VIC, Australia; [c] Department of Thoracic Surgery, St Vincent's Hospital, 55 Victoria Parade, Suite 1, 5th Floor, Melbourne, Fitzroy 3065, VIC, Australia; [d] Eastern Health, Box Hill Hospital, Monash University, 51 Nelson Road, Box Hill 3128, Melbourne, VIC, Australia; [e] Department of Thoracic Surgery, Georgetown University Hospital, 4PHC, 3800 Reservoir Road NW, Washington, DC 20007, USA; [f] Department of Surgery (MMC), The Knox Hospital, Monash University, 262 Mountain Highway, Wantirna 3152, Melbourne, VIC, Australia; [g] The Valley Hospital, Melbourne, VIC, Australia
* Corresponding author.
E-mail address: cliffchoong@hotmail.com

Thorac Surg Clin 23 (2013) 11–16
http://dx.doi.org/10.1016/j.thorsurg.2012.10.009
1547-4127/13/$ – see front matter © 2013 Published by Elsevier Inc.

- Increased pleural permeability (eg, infection)
- Obstruction of pleural lymphatic drainage (eg, malignancy)
- Fluid from other cavities or sites (eg, peritoneal, retroperitoneal, or subarachnoid fluid)
- Rupture of thoracic vessels (eg, hemothorax, chylothorax)

Causes
Transudate (ultrafiltrates of plasma)
- Cardiovascular diseases
  - Congestive cardiac failure
  - Pulmonary embolism (pulmonary embolism can also cause an exudative pleural effusion)
- Infradiaphragmatic
  - Cirrhosis (caused by direct movement of peritoneal fluid through the diaphragm)
  - Peritoneal dialysis
- Other
  - Nephrotic syndrome
  - Hypoalbuminemia from other sources (eg, malnutrition, chronic hepatitis)

Exudate (caused by increased capillary permeability, usually containing protein and cellular debris)
- Infection (most common cause of exudative pleural effusions)
  - Bacterial (pneumonia or systemic infection)
  - Tuberculosis
  - Fungal
  - Viral (respiratory, hepatic, cardiac)
  - Parasitic
- Neoplastic
  - Primary lung cancer
  - Metastatic disease to pleura (most commonly in lung and breast carcinomas)
  - Mesothelioma
- Infradiaphragmatic
  - Pancreatitis
  - Peritonitis
  - Bile duct obstruction
  - Inflammatory bowel disease
  - Intra-abdominal abscess
  - Endoscopic esophageal variceal sclerotherapy
  - Meigs syndrome (ascites and pleural effusion associated with pelvic tumors)
- Immune conditions
  - Rheumatoid arthritis
  - Systemic lupus erythematosus
  - Sjögren syndrome
  - Wegner granulomatosis
  - Ankylosing spondylitis
  - Churg-Strauss syndrome
  - Sarcoidosis

- Medications
  - Amiodarone (antiarrhythmic agent)
  - Bromocriptine (dopamine agonist)
  - Dantrolene (muscle relaxant)
  - Metronidazole (antibiotic)
  - Nitrofurantoin (antibiotic)
  - Procarbazine (chemotherapeutic agent)
- Postoperative
  - Postcardiac surgery
  - Lung transplantation (and also in rejection states)
  - Abdominal surgery (including liver transplantation)
- Other
  - Hemothorax
  - Chylothorax
  - Benign asbestos-related effusion
  - Trapped lung
  - Esophageal rupture
  - Yellow nail syndrome (lower limb lymphedema, nail discoloration, bronchiectasis, sinusitis, and pleural effusion)[5]
  - Amyloidosis

Part II: Approach to Patients with Pleural Effusion

History and examination
The history should be targeted to find the cause of the pleural effusion. Common causes, such as cardiac disease, risk factors for malignancy, and exposure to infection, should be elicited. Other questions, such as the duration of symptoms, whether or not the effusion is recurrent, and the effect of symptoms on patients, will suggest a diagnosis and the appropriate course of management.

Clinical examination should similarly be performed with causes of effusions in mind. The examination of patients will establish whether the effusion is unilateral or bilateral, further aiding diagnosis.

Investigations
Blood tests
- Full blood count including white cell differentiation (can suggest infection or hematological malignancy)
- Biochemistry (eg, renal impairment)
- Liver function tests (for hepatic causes of effusion)
- Albumin
- Lipase
- Lactate dehydrogenase (LDH)
- Blood cultures and serology
- Investigations for autoimmune conditions

Radiological tests
- Chest radiographs: Effusions of greater than 75 mL are visible on chest radiographs.

Effusions can be free flowing or loculated. Lateral decubitus views can confirm the appearance of smaller effusions. A chest radiograph can also show lesions or abnormalities in the lung parenchyma. Chest radiographs have limitations for diagnosis of pleural effusion. Xirouchaki and colleagues[6] reported sensitivity and specificity of 65% and 81%, respectively, in critically ill patients when they compared chest X-ray with bedside ultrasound.[6]

- Ultrasound: Chest ultrasonography is useful in locating small effusions, identifying areas of loculation, and guiding thoracocentesis and pleural biopsies.[2] Bedside ultrasound is becoming a routine part of pleural effusion management because of its accuracy and convenience.
- Computed tomography (CT): Chest CT scans can further identify the causes of the pleural effusion, such as pulmonary, bronchial, or pleural malignancy. It can also characterize the effusion in terms of its size, location, and presence of loculations.
- Positron emission tomography (PET): PET scans are useful in the investigation of malignant pleural effusions.[2]

Thoracocentesis The pleural fluid should always be sampled unless the underlying cause of the effusion is known (eg, heart failure). The morbidity associated with thoracocentesis is low if performed by an experienced operator.[2] If there is any concern about damaging intradiaphragmatic or adjacent structures, such as an enlarged heart, the procedure should be done under ultrasound guidance. Coagulation therapy should be considered in patients with platelets less than 50 000/μL or prolonged clotting time. The most common complications are vagal reactions and pneumothoraces.[2]

The macroscopic appearance of the fluid should be analyzed: straw colored (normal, transudate), milky white (chylothorax), turbid (empyema), bloodstained (trauma, malignant, parapneumonic), food particles (esophageal rupture),[7] and bile in bilothorax. Smell can also be suggestive: putrid in infections caused by anaerobic bacteria and ammoniac in urinothorax.[4]

Laboratory testing of pleural fluid
- Protein: In exudates, the ratio of pleural protein to serum protein is greater than 0.5.[1]
- LDH: In exudates, the ratio of pleural LDH to serum LDH is greater than 0.6.[1]
- pH: The pH is usually 7.45 to 7.55 for transudates and 7.30 to 7.45 for exudates.[2] Pleural fluid pH is the most important laboratory test in the management of parapneumonic

effusions. If the pH is less than 7.2 in patients with parapneumonic effusion, it indicates complicated parapneumonic effusion and necessitates fluid drainage by intercostal catheter insertion or surgery.
- Cholesterol: In exudates, cholesterol is more than 1.16.
- White blood cell and red blood cell count: can indicate the presence of infection or blood, particulary if not visible macroscopically.
- Cultures: micro-organisms in the pleural fluid can be cultured in the case of infection.
- Cytology: The sensitivity for malignancy varies between 40% and 87%.[8]
- Acid-fast bacilli (AFB): Consider tuberculosis polymerase chain reaction if there is lymphocytic pleural effusion.

Fiberoptic bronchoscopy Bronchoscopy can be useful if an endobronchial malignancy is suspected[4] (particularly if patients have symptoms, such as hemoptysis and stridor[2]) because biopsies can be taken at the time of the procedure.

Pleural biopsy Needle biopsy of the pleural is sometimes undertaken and can be performed under local anesthesia. At least 4 biopsy specimens should be taken from the one site.[2,8] A diagnosis of tuberculosis (sensitivity >85%), malignancy (sensitivity of 45%–60%), and amyloidosis can be established.[2] Contraindications include patients with low platelet counts (<50 000 μ/L), skin infections at the site of incision, small effusions (caused by the risk of injury to infradiaphragmatic viscera), and severe respiratory disease (because of the risk of pneumothorax). Complications include bleeding, including hemothorax, pneumothorax, superficial and pleural infection, and injury to the liver or spleen.

Thoracoscopy Thoracoscopy is typically performed under general anesthesia but can be done using a local anesthetic and sedation. It allows for direct visualization of the visceral and parietal pleural, and biopsy of the pleura can be simultaneously performed. Pleurodesis can also be performed for the management of pleural effusions.

Thoracotomy Thoracotomy should only be performed if other diagnostic methods have failed.[2] Thoracotomy is discussed further in the management of pleural effusions.

Management

An algorithm is provided in **Fig. 1**. In 15% of cases, the cause of the effusion cannot be found despite repeated cytology and pleural biopsy.[8] In these

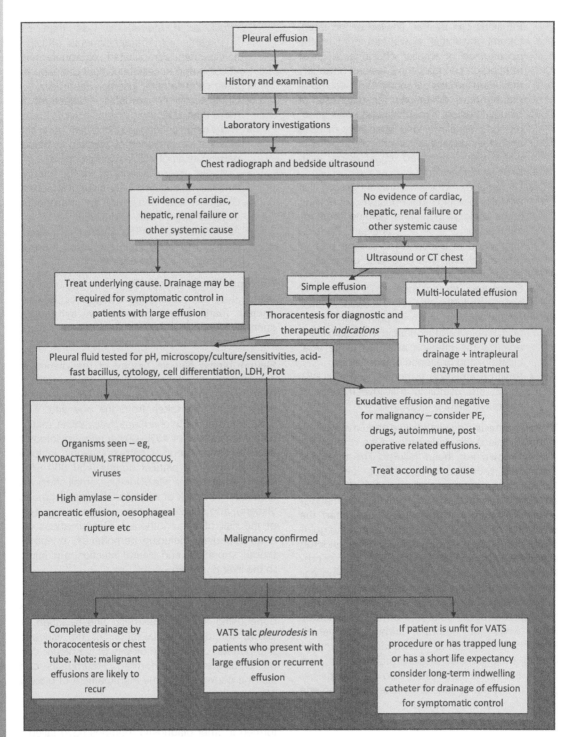

Fig. 1. Algorithm for the diagnosis and management of pleural effusions. *Abbreviations:* PE, pulmonary embolism; Prot, Protein; VATS, video-assisted thoracic surgery.

cases, treatable causes, such as pulmonary embolism, fungal infection, and tuberculosis, should be considered. With continued observation, pleural malignancy will prove to be the cause in many previously undiagnosed effusions.[8]

Benign pleural effusion
Management will depend on the cause of the effusion. Symptomatic relief and diagnosis can be achieved with drainage. In severely loculated effusions or empyema whereby drainage by

thoracocentesis is not possible, either thoraco-scopy or thoracotomy maybe required. Thora-cotomy should be performed if there are dense adhesions and/or a trapped lung seen on thoraco-scopy and whereby it is deemed unsafe by the surgeon to proceed without an open procedure.

Malignant pleural effusion

Malignant cells in pleural fluid (seen on cytology) or the parietal pleura (histopathology from biopsies) indicate disseminated or advanced disease. Sur-vival following diagnosis depends on the type of the underlying malignancy.[9] Metastatic pleural disease is most commonly secondary to lung cancer in men and breast cancer in women.[9]

Most patients presenting with malignant effu-sions are symptomatic. Dyspnea and pleuritic chest pain are the most common presenting symptoms. Patients will often have other systemic symptoms, such as weight loss, anorexia, and malaise. Symptomatic patients should be dis-cussed within a respiratory multidisciplinary team to determine the best management. If patients are asymptomatic with minimal pleural effusion and the tumor type is known, observation may be an appropriate course of action.

Therapeutic thoracocentesis Malignant pleural effusions can be symptomatically managed with thoracocentesis aspiration and drainage of the effusion. However, many of these effusions are likely to recur within weeks of drainage; pleurodesis or indwelling pleural catheter insertion is generally recommended if life expectancy exceeds this time-frame.[10] Thoracocentesis may be appropriate in patients who are too frail for pleurodesis. Indwelling pleural catheter is indicated in patients who are not suitable candidates for video-assisted thoraco-scopic surgery procedures or have been diag-nosed with a trapped lung whereby decortication is considered unsuitable.[11] The amount of fluid drained should be guided by the patient's symp-toms, and if cough or chest discomfort develops, aspiration should be ceased.[12] The rate of drainage of large effusions should be controlled to reduce the risk of reexpansion pulmonary edema.[13]

Pleurodesis Other than patients who are too frail, have a trapped lung, or have a very short life expectancy, pleurodesis is preferable to recurrent thoracocentesis. A sclerosing agent, such as sterile talc, tetracycline, bleomycin, or doxycy-cline, can be used.[12] A diffuse inflammatory reac-tion and fibrin deposition within the pleural space are elicited. In some studies, smaller catheters (10F–14F) have been found to be as effective as conventional large-bore catheters (24F–32F) in the drainage of effusion and pleurodesis.[14] One study found smaller catheters cause less patient discomfort and provide equal efficacy.[15]

In order for pleurodesis to be effective, there needs to be apposition of the visceral and parietal pleura. Incomplete lung expansion can be caused by a trapped lung, pleural loculations, or a per-sistent air leak and needs to be appropriately managed.[12] Suction drainage may be required to promote pleural apposition. A lack of response following pleurodesis is associated with incom-plete lung expansion.[16] Increased pleural fibrino-lytic activity,[17] extensive pleural disease,[18] acidic pleural effusion,[19] and the use of corticosteroids[20] at the time of the pleurodesis can also be associ-ated with failure of pleurodesis.

Pleurodesis can be done either by introducing a talc slurry through an intercostal catheter, or by using aerosolised talc during VATS. The introduc-tion of sclerosing agents can be painful and discomfort can be reduced by administering local anesthetic via the drain before the pleurodesis[12] followed by parenteral narcotics. The authors advise against the use of nonsteroidal antiinflam-matory drugs because of the prevention of an inflammatory response, which is necessary for successful pleurodesis.

Alternatively, pleurodesis can be performed with aerosolized talc, which can be used during thora-coscopy when patients are sedated or under general anesthetic. The advantage of thoraco-scopy is that loculations or adhesions can be visualized and divided, thus aiding in lung reexpan-sion. Also, aerosolized talc can be distributed as it is sprayed throughout the pleural cavity under vision. Pleurodesis during thoracoscopy has a success rate of 77% to 100%,[12] with talc being the preferred agent for this purpose. Thoracoscopy is a safe procedure, with a perioperative mortality of less than 0.5% in several studies.[12] Another substantial advantage with this approach is the decreased risk of pulmonary edema caused by re-expansion being performed with positive pressure under general anesthesia rather than negative pressure if patients are being drained while awake.

Long-term indwelling pleural catheters As briefly mentioned earlier, insertion of a long-term catheter can be useful in controlling recurrent pleural effusions in patients for whom thoracoscopy or pleurodesis is not an appropriate option (eg, frail patients or patients with a trapped lung). The presence of a foreign body within the pleural cavity can stimulate an inflammatory reaction and, thus, encourage spontaneous pleurodesis in some patients.[21] In some patients, drains can be removed after a relatively short period.[12] Patients with indwelling pleural catheters were found to have a shorter length of stay than those who underwent pleurodesis[11,21]; therefore, it may be appropriate for patients for whom hospitalization should be minimized (eg, those with shorter life expectancies). Indwelling catheters should only be used where appropriate expertise and facilities are available.

Parapneumonic effusions and empyema It is crucial to differentiate between simple parapneumonic effusions and complex parapneumonic effusions or empyema because the latter needs drainage with thoracentesis or thoracic surgery.

Empyema is defined by frankly purulent fluid or positive gram stain or culture. Complicated parapneumonic effusion is defined by the presence of loculations (usually found by thoracic ultrasound) or pH less than 7.2. These effusions typically occur in patients who have continued fever and sepsis despite adequate antibiotics.

Complicated pleural effusions may not respond to thoracentesis alone. Intrapleural enzyme treatments have been advocated by some to break the locules and improve pleural fluid drainage. In a blinded randomized controlled trial, intrapleural tissue plasminogen activator and dornase compared with either of these treatments alone improved fluid drainage in patients with parapneumonic pleural effusions. The study found a reduced frequency of surgical referral and duration of hospital stay.[22] In many centers, thoracic surgery remains the main treatment modality in the management of complicated pleural effusions.

REFERENCES

1. Harrison's practice. Available at: http://www.harrisonspractice.com. Accessed July 28, 2012.
2. Garrido VV, Sancho JF, Blasco H, et al. Diagnosis and treatment of pleural effusion. Arch Bronchoneumol 2006;42(7):349–72 [in Spanish].
3. Hooper CE, Lee YC, Maskell NA. Setting up a specialist pleural disease service. Respirology 2010;15:1028–36.
4. Porcel JM, Light RW. Diagnostic approach to pleural effusions in adults. Am Fam Physician 2006;73(7):1211–20.
5. Dhillon SS. Yellow nail syndrome. Am J Respir Crit Care Med 2012;186(6):e10.
6. Xirouchaki N, Magkanas E, Vaporidi K, et al. Lung ultrasound in critically ill patients: comparison with bedside chest radiography. Intensive Care Med 2011;37(9):1488–93.
7. McGrath E, Anderson PB. Diagnosis of pleural effusion: a systematic approach. Am J Crit Care 2011;20(2):119–27.
8. Maskell NA, Butland RJ, A on behalf of the British Thoracic Society Pleural Disease Group. BTS guidelines for the investigation of a unilateral pleural effusion in adults. Thorax 2003;58(Suppl ii):ii8–17.
9. Roberts ME, Neville E, Berrisford RG, et al, on behalf of the BTS Pleural Disease Guideline Group. Management of a malignant pleural effusion: British Thoracic Society pleural disease guideline 2010. Thorax 2010;65(Suppl 2):ii32–40.
10. Light R. Should thoracoscopic talc pleurodesis be the first choice management for malignant effusion? No. Chest 2012;142(1):17–9.
11. Edward TH, Fysh E. Indwelling pleural catheters reduce inpatient days over pleurodesis for malignant pleural effusion. Chest 2012;142(2):394–400.
12. Feller-Kopman D, Walkey A, Berkowitz D, et al. The relationship of pleural pressure to symptom development during therapeutic thoracocentesis. Chest 2006;129:1556–60.
13. Tarver RD, Broderick LS, Conces DJ Jr. Reexpansion pulmonary edema. J Thorac Imaging 1996;11:198–209.
14. Parulekar W, Di Primio G, Matzinger G, et al. Use of small-bore vs large-bore chest tubes for treatment of malignant pleural effusions. Chest 2001;120:19–25.
15. Clementsen P, Evald T, Grode G, et al. Treatment of malignant pleural effusion: pleurodesis using a small percutaneous catheter. A prospective randomized study. Respir Med 1998;92(3):593–6. Accessed on July 28th 2012.
16. Kennedy L, Rusch VW, Strange C, et al. Pleurodesis using talc slurry. Chest 1994;106:242–6.
17. Antony VB, Nasreen N, Mohammad KA, et al. Talc pleurodesis: basic fibroblast growth factor mediates pleural fibrosis. Chest 2004;126:1522–8.
18. Rodriguez-Panadero F, Segado A, Martin JJ, et al. Failure of talc pleurodesis is associated with increased pleural fibrinolysis. Am J Respir Crit Care Med 1995;151:785–90.
19. Heffner JE, Nietert PJ, Barbieri C. Pleural fluid pH as a predictor of pleurodesis failure: analysis of primary data. Chest 2000;117(1):87–95.
20. Xie C, Teixeira LR, McGovern JP. Systemic corticosteroids decrease the effectiveness of talc pleurodesis. Am J Respir Crit Care Med 1998;157:1441–4.
21. Putnam JB Jr, Walsh GL, Swisher SG, et al. Outpatient management of malignant pleural effusion by a chronic indwelling pleural catheter. Ann Thorac Surg 2000;69:369–75.
22. Rahman NM, Maskell NA, West A, et al. Intrapleural use of tissue plasminogen activator and DNase in pleural infection. N Engl J Med 2011;365(6):518–26.

Large-Bore and Small-Bore Chest Tubes
Types, Function, and Placement

David T. Cooke, MD*, Elizabeth A. David, MD

KEYWORDS

- Chest tubes • Small bore • Large bore • Effusions • French

KEY POINTS

- Large-bore chest tubes (LBCTs) are defined as 20 French (Fr) or greater and small-bore chest tubes (SBCTs) are less than 20 Fr.
- Fr is a unit of measurement referring to the outer diameter of the cylindrical tube. A Fr is equivalent to 0.333 mm.
- Chest tubes abide by the physics of Poiseuille's law (for fluids) and the Fanning equation (for air). An increase in the diameter of the tube leads to greater flow of fluid and air.
- With the exception of hemothorax and complex empyema, SBCTs should be considered as first-line pleural drainage therapy. If ineffective, then change to an LBCT or thorascopic surgical therapy should be the next intervention.
- SBCTs are likely ineffective for complex empyema and hemothorax, and LBCTs should be considered standard first-line therapy in that setting.

INTRODUCTION

Pleural tubes or chest tubes are drains that are placed in the pleural space, either surgically or percutaneously, to evacuate abnormal fluid or air. Indications for chest tubes include prophylaxis drainage of air, blood and other fluids after chest surgery (eg, pulmonary resection, esophageal surgery, pleural decortication, and so forth), and therapeutic drainage of pathologic pleural contents such as those found with pneumothorax, hemothorax, empyema, chylothorax, and malignant effusion. This article describes the differences between large-bore chest tubes (LBCTs) and small-bore chest tubes (SBCTs) and characterize the types of chest tubes. The advantages and disadvantages of using each size category, the comparative effectiveness of both tube subsets, and basic techniques and clinical pears for their placement are also discussed.

LBCT
Definition

Chest tubes can be divided into size categories of large bore (≥20 French) and small bore (<20 French). French (Fr) is a unit of measurement first proposed by the French surgical instrument maker Joseph-Frederic-Benoit Charrière in the 1800s. Fr refers to the outer diameter of the cylindrical tube. A Fr is equivalent 0.333 mm. Therefore a 24-Fr chest tube has an outer diameter of 8 mm. Although the outer diameter of a chest tube is consistent, the inner diameter can be variable depending on the thickness of the wall of the chest tube, which varies according to the manufacturer.

Division of Cardiothoracic Surgery, University of California Davis Medical Center, 2221 Stockton Boulevard, Suite 2117, Sacramento, CA 95817, USA
* Corresponding author.
E-mail address: david.cooke@ucdavis.ucdmc.edu

Thorac Surg Clin 23 (2013) 17–24
http://dx.doi.org/10.1016/j.thorsurg.2012.10.006
1547-4127/13/$ – see front matter © 2013 Published by Elsevier Inc.

Two major types of LBCTs are the Argyle type (Covidien, Mansfield, MA) and the Axiom type (Axiom Medical Inc, Torrance, CA). Argyle tubes are made of either polyvinyl chloride (PVC) or silicone; the Axiom tubes are made of silicone. Both tubes contain 5 to 6 drainage holes or eyes extending from the tip (**Fig. 1**). Along the side of each chest tube is a radiopaque line that allows for identification of the chest tube on a plain chest radiograph. The last or most proximal eye is engineered through the radiopaque line so that it can be clearly seen the final hole is in the pleural space (**Fig. 2**). If the clinician chooses to add more holes to the chest tube, then the last additional hole must be cut through the radiopaque line to keep track of the most proximal hole radiographically. Silicone-based chest tubes are softer than the more rigid PVC tubes. Conventional wisdom states that the silicone tube elicits less pain for the patient given the softer structure; however, there have been no randomized trials comparing PVC and silicone tubes to confirm this.

Both chest tube types come in smaller, even small-bore sizes, while maintaining their classic chest tube configuration. They are differentiated from other small-bore tubes such as pigtail catheters in that they are not placed by the Seldinger technique (see later in this article) but by surgical tube thoracostomy like other large-bore tubes. These smaller chest tubes are used frequently in pediatric cardiothoracic surgery, and the appropriate size is based on the weight of the child in kilograms (**Table 1**).

Other types of LBCTs include spiral channel silicone tubes, or Blake drains (Ethicon, Inc, Somerville, NJ). These silicone tubes lack a hollowed out inner lumen, but have a spiral groove that is efficient for draining fluid (**Fig. 3**). The drains are flexible and malleable, and therefore the perception is that they elicit less pain for the patient. The spiral chamber, although efficient for fluid drainage, is often suboptimal for the adequate evacuation of air in the pleural space.

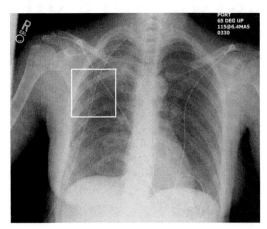

Fig. 2. Proximal hole of a 28-Fr chest tube (*box*) within the pleural space.

Function

Like all cylindrical structures, pleural tubes abide by the physics of Poiseuille's law and the Fanning equation. For liquids, Poiseuille's law states that flow is determined by the viscosity of the liquid, the length of the tube, and pressure changes between the ends of the tube. Flow of gas is determined similarly by the Fanning equation. Chest tubes can drain pleural fluid and air either passively or actively with negative suction generally ranging from -10 to -20 mm Hg.

In both Poisseuille's law and the Fanning equation, small increases in the diameter of the tube lead to greater flow of fluid and air. Therefore, the larger the Fr value of a chest tube, presumably the greater the flow through the tube. However, Fr refers to the outer diameter of a chest tube. As mentioned earlier, the inner diameter can vary depending on the thickness of the tube wall. In addition, patient variables may differ including the consistency and quality of pleural clots and pleural debris, and the presences or absence of free-flowing anatomy of the pleural space, leading to heterogenicity of pleural pressure.

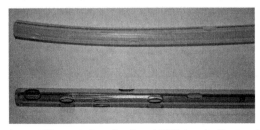

Fig. 1. Silicone Axiom (*top*) and PVC Argyle (*bottom*) 28-Fr chest tubes.

Table 1	
Estimated chest tube size in pediatric patients based on patient weight	
Patient Weight (kg)	**Chest Tube Size (Fr)**
<3	8–10
3–5	10–12
6–10	12–16
11–15	17–22
16–20	22–26
21–30	26–32

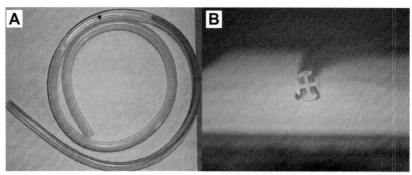

Fig. 3. (*A*) 24-Fr Blake drain. (*B*) Cross-section of a 24-Fr Blake drain.

Indications

The indications for placement of a LBCT are myriad. The British Thoracic Society guidelines give the following indications for chest drain insertion:

- Pneumothorax
- Malignant pleural effusion
- Empyema
- Hemothorax
- Postoperative management of chest cavity

LBCTs are effective for all these indications.[1] However, for stage III fibrinopurulent empyema, the high viscosity and organized characteristics of the effusion make chest tubes ineffective, and surgical lung decortication is necessary. With regard to hemothorax, the Advanced Trauma Life Support Recommendations (ATLS) state that a 36-Fr LBCT should be used for drainage of hemothorax.[2] In a similar setting in postoperative cardiac surgery, Shalli and colleagues[3] surveyed 106 cardiothoracic surgeons and found that 86.8% of the respondents worry that a 20-Fr tube has a higher potential to become clogged with a clot than a larger diameter 36-Fr tube. However, Inaba and colleagues[4] found no difference in the rate of retained hemothorax or even postprocedural pain when comparing LBCTs of 36 to 40 Fr with LBCTs of 28 to 32 Fr in a trauma population requiring open chest tube drainage. Sakopoulos and colleagues[5] found no difference in the need for mediastinal exploration and subsequent additional pleural drainage procedures in patients undergoing cardiac surgery with postprocedure 19-Fr Blake drains compared with traditional LBCTs of 28 to 36 Fr.

SBCTS
Definition

Historically, LBCTs have been used to evacuate pleural fluid and air because of their resistance to

clogging, perhaps at the cost of significant discomfort for the patient both during insertion and while in situ. However, with the development of SBCTs, many pleural conditions can be treated with little difference in clinical efficacy. Typically, SBCTs range from 6 to 19 Fr; 6-Fr tubes are used for pediatric patients. Although randomized trials comparing LBCTs and SBCTs are limited, in recent years, the use of the SBCTs has become more widespread. SBCTs are now routinely used for drainage of pneumothorax, malignant and benign pleural effusion, and empyema.

Types

SBCTs come in many varieties. The most common tubes are pigtail catheters, which curl after removal of a rigid insert (**Fig. 4**). The curved nature of the tube prevents dislodgement of the drain. Pigtails come in varying sizes and are made by several companies including Cook Medical Inc. (Bloomington, IN), C.R. Bard Inc. (Covington, GA), and Boston Scientific Corp. (Natick, MA). Pneumothorax catheter kits are commercially

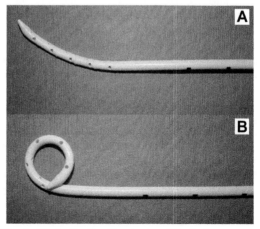

Fig. 4. (*A*) Cook pigtail catheter with rigid insert and (*B*) after removal of insert.

available from Cook Medical ranging from 10 to 14 Fr. They can be placed over trocars or by the Seldinger technique; these kits are designed for simple pneumothoraces.

Trocar catheters from Covidien and Utah Medical Products Inc. (Midvale, UT) are also available. The trocar catheters are single-use devices composed of a sharp or blunt trocar and a clear catheter made of either PVC or silicone. These catheters should be used with caution as acknowledged difficulties and nuances with insertion make the complication rate with these tubes as high as 25%.[6] Previous reports suggest that use of a blunt trocar rather than a sharp trocar may decrease complications; moreover blunt dissection into the chest before tube insertion allows for the safest tube placement when using a trocar chest catheter.[6]

The use of modified single lumen central lines as pleural catheters for both air and fluid drainage has also been described.[7,8] Both groups describe the use of 14-gauge single lumen central venous catheters modified with additional holes in the distal catheter to facilitate drainage. These catheters are placed into the pleural space using a sterile Seldinger technique with good results and lower cost than other pneumothorax kits. It is necessary to use a connector device to connect these single lumen catheters to suction drainage or Heimlich valves; either stopcocks or a Leur-lock connector can be used.

Indwelling pleural catheters are commonly used in the setting of malignant pleural effusions because they result in excellent symptomatic relief of dyspnea for patients and allow for outpatient management.[9] The most common indwelling pleural catheter is the PleurX catheter (Denver Biomaterials Inc, Golden, CO), which is a 15.5-Fr catheter that is tunneled through the skin and then into the pleural space. A one-way valve at the end of the catheter can be connected to vacuum containers to allow for patient-controlled evacuation of fluid. These catheters facilitate drainage of effusions as well as sclerosing therapies, which are helpful in the outpatient management of malignant effusions.

Function

Critics of SBCTs have proposed that smaller tubes are more likely to clog or kink and become nonfunctional, limiting their clinical efficacy. In a study from Duke University comparing 3 sizes and brands of small-bore tubes, flow rates were analyzed using both water and oil.[10] Catheters from Cook, C.R. Bard, and Boston Scientific were compared. There were no significant differences

in flow rates (1.5–2.2 mL/s/s) for 8-Fr tubes between the 3 brands. For the 10-Fr tubes, 2 brands, Bard and Boston Scientific, had significantly faster flow rates than Cook (4.0, 4.1 mL/s/s vs 2.5 mL/s/s, $P<.05$). For the 12-Fr catheters, Bard showed significantly faster flow when compared with the other 2 brands (6.1 mL/s/s vs 4.3, 4.4 mL/s/s, $P<.05$). In this study, Macha and colleagues[10] found no differences in susceptibility to kinking or problems with patency between the brands or sizes. They did find that the presence of a stopcock significantly impaired flow through the catheter regardless of catheter size, which they attributed to the decrease in internal diameter between the standard stopcocks (1.3–1.5 mm) and the tubes themselves (1.7–3.2 mm). The impairment of flow caused by stopcocks is relevant clinically as the smaller tubes are frequently connected with stopcocks to facilitate flushing of the catheter. For this reason, we advocate the use of a large device stopcock rather than a small one to avoid the discrepancy between internal diameters.

In addition to serving as a conduit for drainage of fluid and air, pleural catheters are also used to facilitate pleurodesis in the setting of malignant effusions. Conventional wisdom dictates that SBCTs do not allow for adequate pleurodesis, because tube size limits efficacious delivery of sclerosing therapies. However, it has been demonstrated that tube size does not have any influence on recurrence rates after sclerosis with talc, tetracycline, bleomycin, or interferon in patients with malignant effusions.[11]

Indications

Indications for SBCTs mirror those for LBCTs, including pneumothorax, hemothorax, empyema, malignant pleural effusion, and management of the postoperative chest space. The British Thoracic Society guidelines recommend that small-bore tubes be used where possible because of increased patient comfort except in cases of acute hemothorax.[1] The concern about SBCTs in cases of hemothorax relates to the potential for inadequate drainage resulting in retained hemothorax, and the inability to identify ongoing hemorrhage.[4] Yi and colleagues[12] studied 407 patients who were randomized to chest drainage using either a 16-gauge single lumen central venous catheter (CVC) or conventional chest tubes for traumatic hemothorax. The study found no differences between the groups for indwelling time or severe complications. The identification of progressive hemothorax was possible in the study using changes in pulse rate, blood pressure, and decreased hemoglobin in combination with drainage output. Patients in the study with the CVCs were able to drain more than 1000 mL/h through the CVC. The investigators concluded that the combination of clinical change in vital signs and chest drainage can be used to identify ongoing hemorrhage in patients who have CVCs placed for traumatic hemothorax. Although the support in the medical literature for SBCT use in the setting of hemothorax is compelling, higher powered studies are needed before this practice can be recommended.

The use of SBCTs is increasing as studies continue to demonstrate decreased pain and discomfort, as well as equivalent efficacy for drainage of pneumothorax. In a study of trauma patients with pneumothorax treated with pleural catheters (14 Fr) or chest tubes, Kulvatunyou and colleagues[13] showed no difference in the duration of intubation, the need for mechanical ventilation, or insertion-related complications between the 2 types of tubes. There was a trend toward a higher tube failure rate in the patients who received an SBCT (11% vs 4%, P = .06), but this was not significant. Other series report an 81% success rate for drainage of pneumothorax when using an 8-Fr pleural catheter.[14]

Pneumothorax as an indication for SBCT is intuitive, but their use in empyema is under scrutiny because of concerns about the effectiveness of the tubes in the setting of high viscosity pleural fluid or loculated collections. In 82 patients with effusion (n = 30) or empyema (n = 52) involving 93 SBCTs, Keeling and colleagues[15] found that 19% of patients with empyema went on to require surgical decortication. The patients with empyema were also more likely to require urokinase to maintain tube patency than patients with pleural effusion (51% vs 6%, P<.05).[15] Rahman and colleagues[16] reported no difference in the need for surgery among patients treated with pleural catheters for empyema when tube sizes were compared. They did find an increase in pain scores in patients who received a pleural catheter larger than 20 Fr.[16] In the setting of empyema, the use of SBCTs for definitive therapy should be approached with caution. There should be a low threshold for the placement of additional drains or surgical intervention in patients with empyema who do not demonstrate clinical and radiographic improvement.

COMPARATIVE EFFECTIVENESS OF LARGE-BORE TUBES VERSUS SMALL-BORE TUBES

With advances in radiographic guidance, including computed tomography and ultrasonography, and the relative ease of insertion, the use of SBCTs has become more prevalent. With the increase in the use of SBCTs, it is important to understand the strengths and weaknesses of both types of tubes for various indications. Unfortunately, large multi-institution randomized studies comparing the clinical efficacy, complications, cost, and patient satisfaction with large-bore and small-bore tubes do not exist. Therefore, interpretations of comparisons between the 2 types must be made with care.

Pain

In general, it is thought that SBCTs are less painful both during insertion and while indwelling because there is less disruption and irritation of the intercostal space. However, there is little data to directly determine the effect of tube size on perceived pain. In a study of 52 drains inserted in 44 patients ranging from 12 to 20 Fr, the visual analog scale (VAS) scores for patient pain showed no significant correlation with the size of the tube.[17] In a study of trauma patients receiving chest tubes of 28 to 40 Fr, the VAS scores also showed no correlation with size.[4] Horsley and colleagues'[17] found no difference in the amount of lidocaine for local analgesia used between sizes of tube inserted in their series of SBCTs. From these data, it is difficult to draw a definitive conclusion on superiority of pain with regard to SBCTs and LBCTs.

Complications

As with any invasive procedure, complications can occur during chest tube placement and while they are indwelling. Some of the complications described for chest tubes include malposition, bleeding, infection, pulmonary complications, inadvertent removal, occlusion, or failure of therapy. In their series of trauma patients, Inaba and colleagues[4] found no differences in the overall complication rate, pneumonia after tube placement, infection, or failure of drainage when they compared tube sizes of 28 to 32 Fr versus 36 to 40 Fr. Their overall complication rate was 15.6% and retained hemothorax rate was 11.3%. In a separate study of 122 tubes inserted into 75 patients, a malposition rate of 30% was found for tube sizes of 24 to 32 Fr and use of a trocar was found to be a predicting factor for malposition.[18] In Horsley and colleagues'[17] series with drains of 12 to 20 Fr inserted over a 10-month period, there were no malposition complications using the Seldinger technique for insertion. There was a case of empyema after a drain was inserted for a malignant effusion in 1 patient, but no other infectious complications were reported.[17] The rate of empyema was 4.4% in the trauma patients who underwent placement of tubes of 28 to 40 Fr, with no differences related to the size of tubes.[4] Avoidance of the trocar insertion technique may result in fewer complications related to malpositioning for either large-bore or small-bore tubes. Based on these data, the overall complication rates for large-bore and small-bore tubes seem to be similar.

Effectiveness

In Horsley and colleagues'[17] series, the therapeutic success rate was only 63%, mainly due to drain failure, drain blockage, or dislodgement, but this did not vary by size. The small drains were more successful when used for pneumothorax and malignant or parapneumonic effusions than when used for empyema ($P<.025$).[17] In contrast, in the series of trauma patients who received LBCTs, the procedure success rate was 88.7% when used for traumatic hemothorax.[4] These data suggest that indication for drain placement may be an important factor for decisions about tube size. For empyema it is possible to use SBCTs for drainage and evacuation, but there should be a low threshold for placement of additional drains or proceeding with definitive operative management.

Cost

Tubes that are placed at the bedside using either blunt dissection or insertion or the Seldinger technique cost less than tubes placed under radiographic guidance in a formal interventional radiographic suite. However, there is a risk of malposition when tubes are placed without radiographic guidance, which may add more to the overall cost of treatment. Several factors can contribute to the cost of chest drainage systems including the tubes themselves, suction drainage systems, the use of commercially prepared kits, and the use of reusable instruments from sterile supply. Further studies of cost analysis and effectiveness are needed before definitive conclusions can be drawn based on tube size.

TECHNIQUES FOR PLACEMENT
Placement of LBCTs

Placement of LBCTs is referred to as tube thoracostomy. A tube thoracostomy can be performed at the bedside with minimal patient discomfort if placed properly and with attention to detail. As with any surgical procedure, the first step is logical patient positioning. If, for example, the LBCT is placed in the left pleural space, the left arm is abducted behind the patient's head. A roll is placed behind the left flank, to elevate the patient's side 30° to 45°. Even with normal oxygen saturation, the patient should be given supplemental oxygen. The contralateral arm should be available for intravenous access and blood pressure monitoring. Key external anatomic landmarks are the ipsilateral nipple, tip of the scapula, the costal margin, and the anterior superior iliac spine. LBCTs should be placed anterior to the line of the anterior superior iliac spine or the patient may lie on the chest tube and kink and occlude it when supine; lying on the chest tube can worsen pain. Often LBCTs are placed in the fifth intercostal space in the midaxillary line. If the tube is placed for effusion, it can be placed in a lower intercostal space, but care must be taken to avoid over penetrating through the diaphragm into the peritoneal cavity; the diaphragm, depending on the respiratory cycle, can rise as high as the third intercostal space in some patients.

Local analgesia is achieved with 1% to 2% lidocaine. The appropriate rib is determined and, using a 22-gauge needle, the periosteum is infiltrated with lidocaine. The neurovascular bundle is at the inferior edge of the rib. The needle is passed over the superior edge of the rib while pulling back on the plunger. The needle is advanced until the air or fluid in question is aspirated. The anesthetic is not injected at this point, as it will just disseminate ineffectively into the pleural space. Once air or fluid is aspirated, the needle is slowly withdrawn still pulling back on the plunger until aspiration stops. This point represents the parietal pleura, and liberal injection of anesthetic agent is performed. Afferent nerve fibers are present in the parietal pleura.

An incision of 1 to 2 cm is made over the rib. Using a hemostat, the tissue is dissected using a spreading technique until the pleural space is entered. The pleural defect is then spread widely so that a finger can easily follow the track into the pleural space. Using a finger, the lung is palpated and flimsy adhesions are broken. Thick adhesions should not be bluntly dissected as they can be highly vascular and could result in significant postprocedure bleeding. The LBCT is then inserted using a curved clamp. The clamp is advanced posteriorly and apically. The clamp is released, the tube is inserted, and rotated contralateral to the mediastinum to avoid insertion into the major fissure. It is important to confirm manually that the tube is indeed in the pleural space, because it is easy to mistakenly insert the chest tube extrapleurally, especially in patients with generous adipose tissue (**Fig. 5**).

An additional consideration with SBCTs is the ease with which they can become dislodged, particularly during the placement process. With some kits, it is possible to connect the tube to the suction apparatus or Heimlich valve before placement into the pleural cavity, which can help with patient discomfort during placement as well, because tube manipulation is minimized. This setup is not useful for all patients, and is not recommended when it is necessary to sample pleural fluid for diagnosis.

The ability to place SBCTs with radiographic guidance is a significant advantage over LBCTs. Ultrasonography has been shown to be a safe adjunct to traditional Seldinger or blunt dissection techniques for placement of SBCTs with a low procedure-related complication rate.[19] Transthoracic ultrasonography is also useful for accurate localization and surveillance of pleural effusions, which can not only guide placement but also help guide sclerosing therapies of residual collections.[20] When available, we recommend the use of ultrasonography during placement of SBCTs and for surveillance of the pleural cavity.

SUMMARY

The indications for SBCTs continue to increase, as does their use for upfront drainage of pleural conditions. SBCTs can be as effective as LBCTs for pneumothorax, basic effusions, and simple empyema. with the exception of hemothorax and complex empyema, SBCTs should be considered for first-line drainage therapy. If not effective, then an LBCT or thorascopic surgical therapy should be the next therapeutic intervention. SBCTs are likely ineffective for complex empyema and hemothorax, and LBCTs should be considered standard first-line therapy in that setting.

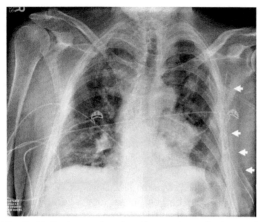

Fig. 5. 28-Fr chest tube placed extrapleurally (*arrows*).

Placement of SBCTs

There is anecdotal consensus that SBCTs are less painful than larger tubes, both on insertion and while indwelling. The decreased pain felt during the indwelling period is largely believed to be secondary to the idea that the catheter is small enough not to disturb the next cephalad rib and impinge on the adjacent intercostal nerve. However, the pain on insertion is largely related to the degree of pressure and force needed to gain entry into the chest and the amount of local analgesia administered during insertion. When we place SBCTs at the bedside, we use generous local 1% to 2% lidocaine based on the weight of the patient in both the subcutaneous space and parietal pleura. Adequate analgesia serves 2 purposes: (1) to decrease irritation caused by the dilators and wires used when inserting a tube with the Seldinger technique; (2) to ensure that the pleural space has been entered by confirming aspiration of air into a syringe filled with local anesthetic. Once adequate analgesia has been established, proceed with tube placement.

SBCTs should be placed at the top of a rib and guided over the rib similar to LBCTs to avoid damage to the neurovascular bundle. SBCTs are typically placed in the second intercostal space along the anterior axillary line, especially when being used for drainage of pneumothorax. However, SBCTs can be placed anywhere into the pleural space. When tubes are being placed under radiographic guidance, care should be taken to place the tube in a position to allow optimal function with attention paid to patient comfort. When placing tubes in a dependent position for fluid drainage, it is important to consider body habitus and position because those factors may affect patient comfort and tube patency.

REFERENCES

1. Laws D, Neville E, Duffy J, Pleural Diseases Group, Standards of Care Committee, British Thoracic Society. BTS guidelines for the insertion of a chest drain. Thorax 2003;58(Suppl 2):ii53–9.
2. American College of Surgeons, Committee on Trauma. ATLS: advanced trauma life support for doctors. 8th edition. Chicago: American College of Surgeons; 2008.
3. Shalli SS, Saeed D, Fukamachi K, et al. Chest tube selection in cardiac and thoracic surgery: a survey of chest tube-related complications and their management. J Card Surg 2009;24:503–9.
4. Inaba K, Lestenberger T, Recinos G, et al. Does size matter? A prospective analysis of 29-32 versus

36-40 French chest tube size in trauma. J Trauma 2012;72:422–7.

5. Sakopoulos AG, Hurwitz AS, Suda RW, et al. Efficacy of Blake drains for mediastinal and pleural drainage following cardiac operations. J Card Surg 2005;20:574–7.

6. Ortner CM, Ruetzler K, Schaumann N, et al. Evaluation of performance of two different chest tubes with either a sharp or a blunt tip for thoracostomy in 100 human cadavers. Scand J Trauma Resusc Emerg Med 2012;20:10.

7. Marshall MB. Modified central line for pneumothorax. Ann Thorac Surg 2006;82(4):1543–4.

8. Ishibashi H, Ohta S, Hirose M. Modified central venous catheter for pneumothorax. Gen Thorac Cardiovasc Surg 2008;56(6):309–10.

9. Davies HE, Mishra EK, Kahan BC, et al. Effect of an indwelling pleural catheter vs chest tube and talc pleurodesis for relieving dyspnea in patients with malignant pleural effusion: the TIME2 randomized controlled trial. JAMA 2012;307(22):2383–9.

10. Macha DB, Thomas J, Nelson RC. Pigtail catheters used for percutaneous fluid drainage: comparison of performance characteristics. Radiology 2006; 238(3):1057–63.

11. Parulekar W, Di Primio G, Matzinger F, et al. Use of small-bore vs large-bore chest tubes for treatment of malignant pleural effusions. Chest 2001;120(1):19–25.

12. Yi JH, Liu HB, Zhang M, et al. Management of traumatic hemothorax by closed thoracic drainage using a central venous catheter. J Zhejiang Univ Sci B 2012;13(1):43–8.

13. Kulvatunyou N, Vijayasekaran A, Hansen A, et al. Two-year experience of using pigtail catheters to treat traumatic pneumothorax: a changing trend. J Trauma 2011;71(5):1104–7 [discussion: 1107].

14. Gammie JS, Banks MC, Fuhrman CR, et al. The pigtail catheter for pleural drainage: a less invasive alternative to tube thoracostomy. JSLS 1999;3(1): 57–61.

15. Keeling AN, Leong S, Logan PM, et al. Empyema and effusion: outcome of image-guided small-bore catheter drainage. Cardiovasc Intervent Radiol 2008;31(1):135–41.

16. Rahman NM, Maskell NA, Davies CW, et al. The relationship between chest tube size and clinical outcome in pleural infection. Chest 2010;137(3): 536–43.

17. Horsley A, Jones L, White J, et al. Efficacy and complications of small-bore, wire-guided chest drains. Chest 2006;130(6):1857–63.

18. Remérand F, Luce V, Badachi Y, et al. Incidence of chest tube malposition in the critically ill: a prospective computed tomography study. Anesthesiology 2007;106(6):1112–9.

19. Liu YH, Lin YC, Liang SJ, et al. Ultrasound-guided pigtail catheters for drainage of various pleural diseases. Am J Emerg Med 2010;28(8): 915–21.

20. Sartori S, Tombesi P, Tassinari D, et al. Sonographically guided small-bore chest tubes and sonographic monitoring for rapid sclerotherapy of recurrent malignant pleural effusions. J Ultrasound Med 2004;23(9):1171–6.

Causes and Management of Common Benign Pleural Effusions

Rajesh Thomas, MBBS, FRACP[a],
Y.C. Gary Lee, MBChB, PhD, FRACP, FRCP[a,b],*

KEYWORDS

- Pleural • Effusion • Empyema • Pleurodesis • Malignant • Parapneumonic • Chylothorax
- Mesothelioma

KEY POINTS

- Benign pleural effusions have diverse causes and manifestations, which often makes their diagnosis and management challenging. They are twice as common as malignant effusions.
- Differentiating effusions as a transudate or exudate is helpful in directing investigations and management. Extensive investigations may not be necessary in transudative effusions.
- Congestive heart failure and hepatic hydrothorax are the commonest causes for transudative effusion. Treatments are directed at the underlying cause, although a more specialized approach may be required in refractory cases.
- Parapneumonic effusions secondary to bacterial infections and tuberculous effusions (in endemic regions) are the commonest type of benign exudative effusions. Other common causes include pulmonary embolism, drugs, collagen vascular diseases, or they may occur after cardiac surgery. More extensive diagnostic evaluation including detailed clinical history, appropriate imaging and pleural sampling, and a tailored management approach are often required in exudative effusions.

INTRODUCTION

Pleural effusion is a common cause of morbidity worldwide; its incidence and causes vary depending on the population studied. An estimated 1 million patients suffer from a pleural effusion annually in the United States alone.[1]

Pleural effusions can arise from diseases of the pleura or extrapleural, particularly cardiopulmonary, though anatomical variations are common disorders. More than 90% of all effusions in developed countries are caused by congestive heart failure (CHF), malignancy, pneumonia, and pulmonary embolism.[2] Tuberculosis (TB) is a common cause of pleural effusions in endemic regions.

Although malignancy is always a concern in patients presenting with a pleural effusion, more than 60 benign causes have been described.[3] Benign pleural effusions are at least twice as common as malignant ones in most epidemiologic

Conflict of interests declaration: Professor Lee has received honoraria as an advisor to CareFusion and Sequana Medical. He was a coinvestigator of the MIST-2 and TIME-2 trials, which received funding or equipment support from Roche and Rocket Medical. Professor Lee receives research funding from the New South Wales Dust Disease Board, Cancer Council of Western Australia, and Sir Charles Gairdner Research Advisory Committee.
 a Department of Respiratory Medicine, Sir Charles Gairdner Hospital, Hospital avenue Perth, Western Australia 6009, Australia; b Centre for Asthma, Allergy and Respiratory Research, School of Medicine & Pharmacology, University of Western Australia, Perth, Western Australia 6009, Australia
* Corresponding author. University Department of Medicine, Sir Charles Gairdner Hospital, 4/F, G Block, Perth, Western Australia 6009, Australia.
E-mail address: gary.lee@uwa.edu.au

Thorac Surg Clin 23 (2013) 25–42
http://dx.doi.org/10.1016/j.thorsurg.2012.10.004
1547-4127/13/$ – see front matter © 2013 Elsevier Inc. All rights reserved.

series (**Table 1**). The diverse causes and manifestations of benign effusions make them common diagnostic challenges. This article describes the clinical approach to common benign pleural effusions.

PATHOPHYSIOLOGY OF PLEURAL EFFUSION FORMATION

The normal physiologic pleural fluid is a transudate with an estimated volume of 0.1 to 0.2 mL/kg body weight.[4] Excessive accumulation of pleural fluid develops when the rate of fluid formation exceeds its drainage capacity. This situation can result from increased pleural fluid formation or decreased fluid absorption, or often both.[5]

LIGHT'S CRITERIA

Given the many causes of pleural effusions, conventionally the workup of pleural effusions begins by broadly triaging them as transudates and exudates. The differential diagnosis and pathophysiology of transudates and exudates are different, as is often the management.

Transudates arise from imbalances between the hydrostatic and/or oncotic pressures, which result in fluid extravasation and accumulation in the pleural cavity.[6] The underlying pleura and the vascular permeability to proteins remain normal. In contrast, most exudative effusions develop as a result of vascular hyperpermeability and plasma leak, usually a manifestation of malignant or inflammatory disorders. The underlying disease(s) may also impair fluid drainage via the stomata on the parietal pleura or the downstream lymphatic channels.

The Light's criteria are commonly used to distinguish between transudative and exudative pleural effusions.[7] An exudative pleural effusion is one that fulfills 1 or more of the following 3 criteria, whereas a transudate is one that meets none[7]:

1. Pleural fluid/serum protein ratio greater than 0.5
2. Pleural fluid/serum lactate dehydrogenase (LDH) ratio greater than 0.6
3. Pleural fluid LDH greater than two-thirds the upper limit of normal for serum LDH

The Light's criteria can identify an exudative effusion with a sensitivity of 98% and specificity of 74%,[8] and is better than other parameters proposed to date. The Light's criteria are designed to be conservative and to rather overcall effusions as exudates than to misclassify exudates as transudates. False-positive and false-negative results do occur, and clinical judgment must be exercised in the interpretation of results. One common example of false exudate occurs in patients with CHF receiving diuretics whose pleural fluid often has a protein level in the exudative range.[9] Clinicians may also be misguided by separation of effusion into a transudate or exudate if there are concurrent (and opposing) causes of the effusion (eg, concomitant pleural malignancy and CHF).

Triaging effusions into transudates or exudates does not provide a diagnosis. An increasing number of disease-specific biomarkers are now available to help define the cause of an effusion.[10]

Nonetheless, defining a pleural effusion as a transudate or exudate remains helpful in directing investigations in most cases. Extensive investigations are unnecessary in cases of transudative effusions and management is primarily directed at treating the underlying cause (eg, CHF). An exudate often demands a more extensive diagnostic evaluation, and management is directed toward control of the effusion and treatment of the underlying cause.[11]

TRANSUDATIVE PLEURAL EFFUSIONS

Overall, transudative pleural effusions are more common than exudates in unselected patient populations. CHF and hepatic hydrothorax are the commonest causes for a transudative effusion. Uncommon causes include nephrotic syndrome, amyloidosis, urinothorax, peritoneal dialysis, and hypothyroidism (**Table 2**).[3,11]

CHF

CHF accounts for almost half of all pleural effusions in many series.[2,12]

Table 1 Estimated annual incidence of common benign pleural effusions in the United States	
Type of Effusion	**Annual Incidence**
CHF effusions	500,000
Parapneumonic effusion (including empyema)	300,000
Pulmonary emboli-related effusions	150,000
Viral pleuritis	100,000
Postcoronary artery bypass surgery effusions	60,000
Hepatic hydrothorax	50,000
Collagen vascular disease-related effusions	6000
TB pleuritis	2500
Asbestos-related pleural effusions	2000

Data from Light RW. Pleural diseases. 4th edition. Philadelphia: Lippincott Williams & Wilkins; 2001.

Table 2
Common benign pleural effusions

	Common Causes	Less Common Causes
Transudative effusions	CHF Liver cirrhosis Peritoneal dialysis fluid Hypoalbuminemia	Pericardial disease[a] Nephrotic syndrome Urinothorax Myxoedema Central venous occlusion Atelectasis/trapped lung Amyloidosis[a]

Exudative effusions	Infections
	  Bacterial
	  TB
	Postsurgical effusions
	  Postcardiac injury syndrome
	  Postcoronary artery bypass effusion
	Pulmonary embolism
	Drug-induced
	Collagen vascular diseases
	Asbestos-related effusions
		Infections
		  Fungal
		  Viral
		  Parasitic
		  Actinomycosis
		  Nocardiosis
		Gastrointestinal/Abdominal diseases
		  Reactive effusion or spread from
		    subphrenic, liver, or splenic abscesses
		  Esophageal perforation
		  Pancreatitis
		Chylothorax
		Hemothorax
		Meigs syndrome
		Yellow nail syndrome

[a] Can be transudative or exudative.
Data from Light RW, Lee YG, editors. Textbook of pleural diseases. 2nd edition. London: Hodder Arnold; 2008; and Hooper C, Lee YC, Maskell N, et al. Investigation of a unilateral pleural effusion in adults: British Thoracic Society Pleural Disease Guideline 2010. Thorax 2010;65(Suppl 2):ii4–17.

Pathophysiology

Increased hydrostatic pressure from CHF alters the equilibrium of the Starling forces and results in increased fluid accumulation in the lung interstitium. If the lymphatic drainage of the lung is saturated, the excess fluid can drain into the pleural space. Pleural effusion becomes detectable only when the fluid reaching the pleural cavity exceeds its drainage capacity.[13] Hence, the finding of pleural effusion in CHF usually indicates significant fluid overload. Although uncommon, pleural effusions may develop in patients with right heart failure.[14]

Clinical manifestation

Signs and symptoms are predominantly those of CHF. Pleuritic pain is rare. Pleural effusions can be seen on chest radiographs of as many as two-thirds of patients with CHF and are bilateral in ~50% patients. Unilateral effusions are more commonly right-sided.[15,16]

The effusions are usually small to medium in size, and are asymptomatic findings on chest radiographs. If there are no other radiographic signs of CHF (eg, cardiomegaly) or the effusion is unilateral (or significantly asymmetrical), alternative causes should be considered.

The British Thoracic Society Pleural Disease Guidelines suggest that in a patient with a typical history of CHF and bilateral symmetric effusions with no suspicion of other concurrent causes, it is reasonable to treat the effusion without a diagnostic thoracentesis. A diagnostic thoracentesis is indicated only if atypical features exist.[11]

If the fluid is sampled, it should be a transudate. However, a proportion of CHF pleural effusions may meet the Light's criteria as an exudate, particularly with diuretic treatment or after repeated thoracenteses. Some investigators suggest that in such patients, the fluid can be reclassified as a transudate if the difference between the serum and pleural fluid protein level is greater than 3.1 g/dL.[17]

Measurement of pleural fluid N-terminal pro-brain natriuretic peptide (NTpro-BNP) is a reliable marker for diagnosing CHF effusion, especially in those misclassified as exudates by the Light's criteria (**Fig. 1**).[18] The best cutoff value varied among studies, although most use around 1500 pg/mL. Pleural fluid NTpro-BNP is superior to BNP in establishing the diagnosis of CHF effusions.[18]

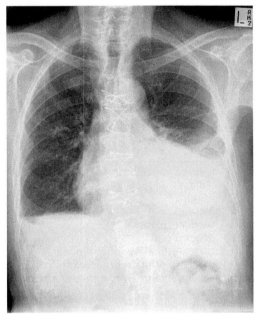

Fig. 1. Measurement of pleural fluid NTpro-BNP is a reliable marker for diagnosing CHF effusion that is misclassified as exudate by the Light's criteria. Chest radiograph of a man with history of ischemic heart disease and previous coronary artery bypass graft, showing bilateral, predominantly left-sided pleural effusion and cardiomegaly. Pleural fluid was border-line exudate (increased protein and low LDH level) by Light's criteria but showed high NTpro-BNP of more than 7000 ng/L (normal <1500 ng/L), which is consistent with effusion secondary to heart failure, thus avoiding unnecessary investigations.

Management

Treatment is directed at optimizing management of heart failure. If the effusion fails to resolve with treatment of heart failure, alternative (or concomitant) causes should be kept in mind. Therapeutic thoracentesis may benefit dyspneic patients with a large effusion. In patients with a refractory and symptomatic effusion despite optimal medical therapy, pleurodesis can be considered. Rarely, an indwelling pleural catheter (IPC) or pleuroperitoneal shunt can be used.[19]

Other Cardiac Disease-Related Effusions

Pericardial disease

Pathophysiology Pericardial diseases can cause transudative or exudative effusions, depending on the pericardial disease or presence of heart failure. It is likely that effusions develop as an extension of pericardial inflammation to the adjacent pleura.[20] Simultaneous involvement of the pericardium and left pleura by the same underlying process (eg, TB or malignancy) can sometimes occur.

Clinical manifestation Most effusions related to pericardial disease are left-sided (particularly with acute pericarditis) or bilateral.[20] Unlike CHF, patients with pericarditis usually have pleuritic chest pain and dyspnea. Clinical signs of pericarditis or pericardial tamponade may be present.

Management Management should focus on treating the pericardial disease. The pleural effusion usually does not require specific treatment unless it is large and causing dyspnea.

Hepatic Hydrothorax

Hepatic hydrothorax is defined as a pleural effusion in a patient with liver cirrhosis and no other causes of effusion. It affects ~6% of patients with cirrhosis; many (>80%), but not all, have ascites.[21] The effusion is usually unilateral and right-sided (~85%), although bilateral or rarely left-sided effusions can occur.[22,23]

Pathophysiology

The exact pathogenesis is debated. Decreased plasma oncotic pressure from hypoalbuminemia contributes to fluid formation. The most accepted theory is that ascitic fluid leaks from the peritoneal cavity into the pleural space through small diaphragmatic defects.[24,25] The negative intrapleural pressure relative to the intraperitoneal pressure helps drive fluid into the pleural pace.

Clinical manifestation

Symptoms from the underlying cirrhosis and ascites predominate. The degree of dyspnea depends on the size of the effusion. Hepatic hydrothorax should be suspected in any patient with liver cirrhosis and a (particularly right-sided) pleural effusion, even without ascites.

The effusion is usually a transudate.[26] Other (eg, cardiopulmonary) causes for an effusion may need to be ruled out whenever clinically appropriate.[27]

Spontaneous bacterial empyema, defined as spontaneous infection of preexisting hepatic hydrothorax, can occur and has a high mortality (~20%). Pleural fluid polymorphonuclear cell count usually exceeds 500 cells/mL. Usual organisms isolated include *Escherichia coli*, *Streptococcus* species, *Enterococci*, and *Klebsiella*.[28]

Rarely, chylothorax may be seen secondary to liver cirrhosis[29,30] and results from transdiaphragmatic passage of chylous ascites.[30]

Management

Treating recurrent hepatic hydrothorax can be difficult. Initial therapy is primarily directed toward management of the underlying liver cirrhosis and portal hypertension. The definitive therapy for hepatic hydrothorax remains liver transplantation or transjugular intrahepatic portal systemic shunt (TIPS).[31] TIPS controls hepatic hydrothorax in up to 80% of patients by reducing portal pressure and the increased hepatic sinusoidal pressure that causes ascites[32] and is useful as a bridge to transplantation.[33]

Pleural fluid control and symptomatic relief are important for patients awaiting transplantation or TIPS and those unsuitable for these treatments. Dietary sodium restriction and diuretics should be tried but are often insufficient to control fluid accumulation.[34] Repeated thoracentesis can be considered, although frequent pleural drainage may hasten protein and electrolyte depletion and pose infection and bleeding risks, because coagulopathy is common in these patients.

Pleurodesis can be attempted but rapid transdiaphragmatic migration of fluid has been blamed for the high failure rate. Use of continuous positive pressure ventilation to reduce pleural influx of ascitic fluid after talc pleurodesis has been reported.[35] Thoracoscopic pleurodesis and closure of diaphragmatic defects in the same setting have been attempted.[36] IPCs have been used with some success.[37]

EXUDATIVE PLEURAL EFFUSIONS
Parapneumonic Effusions and Empyema

Parapneumonic effusions usually complicate bacterial pneumonia and are the commonest exudative pleural effusions. More than 1 million patients are hospitalized for community-acquired pneumonia annually in the United States[38]; almost 50% of these patients develop a pleural effusion.[39] Those patients with pneumonia who developed a parapneumonic effusion have a higher morbidity and mortality (~22%) compared with those without an effusion.[40,41]

Pathophysiology
Effusions associated with pneumonia include simple and complicated parapneumonic effusions, and empyemas. Simple parapneumonic effusions arise from reactive vascular hyperpermeability associated with pleural inflammation accompanying the underlying pneumonia. These effusions are usually small and sterile.[39]

A complicated parapneumonic effusion usually indicates an infected pleural space. It is characterized by pleural fluid neutrophilia, low pleural fluid pH and glucose, high LDH level, and fibrinous septations causing multiple loculations within the pleural space. Empyema is characterized by presence of frank pus or bacteria within the pleural space. Pleural infection is often defined in clinical trials to encompass both complicated parapneumonic effusion and empyema.

Bacteriology
Pleural infection is often secondary to an underlying pneumonic process. However, a sizable subgroup of patients develop pleural infection without evidence of pneumonia, even on computed tomography (CT). The disparity between common organisms of pneumonia and those of pleural infection also support alternative causes of some empyemas. *Streptococcus milleri* in particular is a group of oral commensals that have been shown to be the most common bacterial cause of community-acquired empyema[42]; yet pneumonia with *Streptococcus milleri* is rare.

It is important to define pleural infections as community-acquired or hospital-acquired, because their bacteriology and optimal antimicrobial therapy differ. Common organisms (**Table 3**) in community-acquired pleural infection include streptococci (especially *Streptococcus intermedius* or *Streptococcus pneumoniae*), which account for ~50% of cases, anaerobic bacteria (~25% of cases), and staphyloccoci and gram-negative organisms (~10% of cases).[42] Hospital-acquired empyemas are most commonly caused by *Staphylococcus aureus* (~35% of cases), especially methicillin-resistant *Staphylococcus aureus*, and gram-negative organisms (~25%).

Clinical manifestation
Parapneumonic effusion should be suspected in all patients with pneumonia who develop a pleural effusion, especially when patients lack clinical response despite antimicrobial therapy. Chronic alcohol abuse, intravenous drug use, and younger (<60 years) age are independent predictors for development of pleural infection in pneumonic patients.[43,44]

Most patients present with fever, productive cough, chest pain, leukocytosis, and increased inflammatory markers. Patients with anaerobic bacterial pleural infections can present with a subacute illness with nonspecific constitutional symptoms.[45]

Management
A high index of clinical suspicion is necessary for early detection of simple parapneumonic effusions and may avoid their progression to pleural infection.[42] A small or moderate effusion can be difficult to detect on a chest radiograph, particularly in the presence of lung consolidation. Pleural ultrasonography is a more sensitive test for small effusions and for pleural septations. A pleural-phase CT scan is useful particularly to differentiate between empyema and a lung abscess. A characteristic split pleura sign is often seen in empyema as a result of enhancement of the parietal and visceral pleurae separated by a pleural collection.[39]

Table 3
Bacteriology of community-acquired and hospital-acquired pleural infection (UK data)[a]

Community-Acquired Isolates N = 336	Hospital-Acquired N = 60
Streptococci: 176 (52%)	*Staphylococcus aureus*: 21 (35%)
Streptococcus intermedius (*milleri* group): 80 (24%)	Methicillin-sensitive: 6 (10%)
Streptococcus pneumoniae: 71 (21%)	Methicillin-resistant: 15 (25%)
Other streptococcal species: 25 (7%)	Gram-negative bacteria: 14 (23.3%)
Anaerobes: 67 (20%)	*Escherichia coli, Pseudomonas aeruginosa*,
Fusobacterium, Bacteroides, and	and other coliforms
Prevotella spp	Streptococci: 11 (18.3%)
Staphylococcus aureus: 35 (10.4%)	*Streptococcus intermedius* (*milleri*) group,
Methicillin-sensitive: 27 (8%) and	*Streptococcus pneumonia*, and other
methicillin-resistant *Staphylococcus*	streptococcal species
aureus: 7 (2%)	*Enterococcus* spp: 7 (12%)
Gram-negative bacteria: 29 (8.6%)	Anaerobes: 5 (8.3%)
Escherichia coli, Proteus, and *Enterobacter*	

[a] Only most common organisms are included in the table. Please refer to original publication for complete list of bacteria.
Data from Maskell NA, Batt S, Hedley EL, et al. The bacteriology of pleural infection by genetic and standard methods and its mortality significance. Am J Respir Crit Care Med 2006;174:817–23.

Parapneumonic effusion in the presence of fever and increased inflammatory markers requires prompt pleural drainage. Multiple loculations often form with time and can impair fluid drainage. Pleural fluid should be sampled if there is clinical suspicion of pleural infection.[39]

Treatment of pleural infections comprises 2 cardinal principles: appropriate antibiotics and early pleural drainage. Antibiotics and tube drainage are sufficient treatment in many patients; however, up to 30% of patients may require additional intrapleural therapy or surgery.[41,46]

Antibiotics

Choice of the appropriate antibiotic depends on local bacterial resistance pattern and the causative organisms. Up to 40% of patients with empyema have no organisms cultured; clinicians have to choose antimicrobials based on the local bacteriology. In hospital-acquired empyema, a broader antibiotic coverage is needed.[42]

Drainage

Simple parapneumonic effusions are sterile and usually require no treatment other than appropriate antibiotics for the pneumonia. Complicated parapneumonic effusions and empyemas usually require drainage for resolution.

Initial management usually involves placement of an intercostal tube. Image guidance is strongly encouraged to direct optimal tube placement, especially for multiloculated effusions. Large clinical series have shown no difference in outcome of patients managed with large tubes or small-bore (≤16 F) catheters. The latter is usually inserted by the Seldinger technique using image guidance and is associated with fewer complications and less pain.[47,48]

For patients who fail to respond clinically (ongoing fever and raised infection markers) to antibiotics and chest tube drainage, further imaging (eg, CT) is necessary to exclude other ongoing sources of sepsis (eg, lung abscess) and to delineate any significant residual pleural collections. If the latter is deemed the source for ongoing infection, there are several options to enhance fluid evacuation. If there are only 1 or 2 residual collections, placement of a second chest tube under imaging guidance is often adequate. In cases of multiple loculations, intrapleural therapy or surgery is recommended.

Intrapleural fibrinolysis alone using streptokinase and tissue plasminogen activator (tPA) have failed to show a benefit in randomized studies, namely MIST-1 (Multi-Center Intrapleural Sepsis Trial) and MIST-2, respectively.[41,48] However, the combined use of intrapleural tPA and deoxyribonuclease (DNase) in MIST-2 significantly improved evacuation of pleural infection, shortened hospitalization, and successfully treated 95% of patients without needing surgery (**Fig. 2**).[49]

Surgery should be considered if sepsis persists despite appropriate therapy and drainage.[50] Video-assisted thoracoscopic surgery is usually the surgical procedure of choice and is successful in ~80% of patients. Conversion to thoracostomy is needed in the remaining patients, especially those with advanced empyema and a thick visceral peel prohibiting full lung expansion.[51]

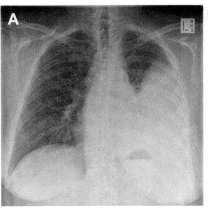
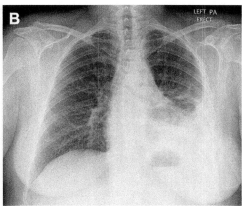

Fig. 2. Successful use of intrapleural tPA-DNase in pleural infection with loculated fluid. Serial radiographs show radiological improvement of effusion after successful treatment with small-bore chest tube and tPA-DNase. (*A*) Loculated effusion that persists despite insertion of small-bore chest tube in a young patient with pleural infection. (*B*) Significant radiological improvement (which was also associated with significant clinical improvement) seen 3 days after intrapleural instillation of tPA-DNase.

Use of surgery as first-line treatment is practiced in many centers worldwide. Five randomized trials (3 in pediatric and 2 adults) have failed to show a significant advantage of this practice.[52] The only benefit shown was a slightly shorter hospital stay (12 vs 8 days), without differences in mortality.[53,54] This finding has to be balanced between higher surgical morbidity (especially pain) and costs.[55,56] Residual pleural opacity on imaging resolves over time (usually within weeks), as shown in 2 clinical series (**Fig. 3**).[41,57] If the patient's infection signs are adequately treated/controlled with antibiotics and drainage, there is no need to subject them to surgical debridement or decortications.[39] This strategy is akin to management of residual pneumonic changes in patients adequately treated for their infection.

For further reading; refer to Davies and colleagues.[50]

Tuberculous Pleural Effusion

Pleural effusion is one of the commonest extrapulmonary manifestations of TB. In endemic countries, TB pleuritis complicates more than 25% of patients with TB and is one of the commonest causes of exudative pleural effusions.[58] However, in the United States, only one of 30 patients with TB develops a pleural effusion.[59] A higher incidence of TB pleural effusion is seen in patients with human immunodeficiency virus who developed TB.[60]

Pathophysiology

Tuberculous pleuritis can develop from a primary mycobacterial infection that was acquired in the preceding months or after reactivation of latent tuberculous infection.[39] In developed countries,

reactivation of latent TB is believed to be the commonest cause of tuberculous pleuritis.[61]

Tuberculous pleuritis develops after rupture into the pleural space of a subpleural lung parenchymal caseous focus followed by a delayed hypersensitivity reaction to the mycobacterial protein.[62] The mycobacterial load is often low and explains why the pleural fluid/tissue culture for mycobacteria has a poor yield.[63]

Clinical manifestation

Patients may present with an acute febrile illness associated with pleuritic chest pain and cough, or insidiously with dyspnea and constitutional symptoms (eg, weight loss, night sweat, and malaise).[39]

Tuberculous effusions are usually unilateral but can vary in sizes.[64] In some series, most (86%) patients show lung parenchymal abnormalities on CT scans, and 56% of patients show evidence of active pulmonary TB.[65] The pleural fluid is usually an exudate with a high protein level and low glucose level and is predominantly lymphocytic (ie, lymphocytes >50% of the total leukocytes in the fluid) in more than 90% of cases.[64]

Evidence of mycobacterium in sputum, pleural fluid, or pleural biopsy specimens, or evidence of caseating granulomas on pleural biopsy specimen, provides the diagnosis of tuberculous pleuritis. In 1 study, 52% of patients had a positive sputum culture even in the absence of lung parenchymal infiltrates on chest radiograph, although the results have never been replicated.[66] Pleural fluid smears are usually negative for mycobacteria and less than 40% of immunocompetent patients have a positive yield on pleural fluid culture, although the yield is higher in immunocompromised hosts.[64] Because the pleura is diffusely involved in

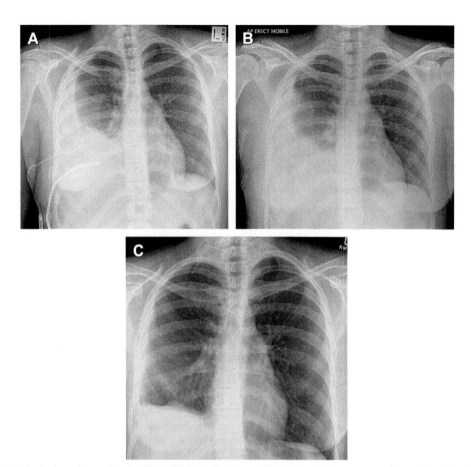

Fig. 3. Residual pleural opacity usually resolves with time without need for surgery after systemic infection is controlled. Serial radiographs show radiological improvement of effusion and residual pleural opacity after successful treatment with antibiotics and small-bore chest tube in a 19-year-old who developed pleural infection after appendicectomy. (*A*) Persistent pleural effusion despite chest tube drainage. However, the patient's fever and inflammatory markers all settled with antibiotics. (*B*) Chest tubes were removed and the patient discharged with antibiotics. Residual pleural opacity (despite complete clinical response and resolution of previously increased inflammatory markers) after removal of chest tube. (*C*) Spontaneous improvement of pleural thickening over a period of 1 month.

tuberculous effusion, blind pleural biopsy has a yield of ~80% on histopathology alone and ~90% if, in addition, the pleural tissue is subjected to mycobacterial culture.[64] Thoracoscopic biopsy is useful to clinch the diagnosis (**Fig. 4**).[67]

Pleural fluid adenosine deaminase (ADA) has high sensitivity and specificity (both >90%) for diagnosing TB effusions.[68] In many resource-limited regions, a positive ADA in the compatible clinical picture of tuberculous pleural effusion is now used to decide on initiation of therapy. However, increased pleural fluid ADA is also found in empyema and some cases of cancer or connective tissue disorders. In nonendemic areas, a low ADA level has a high negative predictive value.

Management

TB pleural effusions usually resolve spontaneously. Antituberculous therapy should still be

initiated, because up to 65% of untreated patients with tuberculous effusions develop active TB (usually within 5 years).[69]

Patients should be treated with standard antimycobacterial therapy, and the effusion usually resolves within weeks.[70] Pleural symptoms (pain and effusion) may persist occasionally, and some patients (up to 16%) may suffer a paradoxic worsening of the effusion.[71] Therapeutic drainage or a short course of systemic corticosteroids may relieve symptoms, although their routine use is not recommended, because neither alters long-term outcome, especially the incidence of fibrothorax.[72]

Pulmonary Embolism

Pulmonary embolism is a common cause of pleural effusion and may be seen in almost half

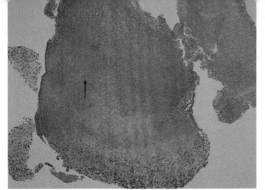

Fig. 4. Closed or thoracoscopic pleural biopsy has a high yield for rapid diagnosis of tuberculous pleural effusion because the pleura is diffusely involved. Histopathology of thoracoscopic pleural biopsy in a young female patient with undiagnosed pleural effusion showing a necrotizing granuloma composed of a central zone of caseous necrosis (*black arrow*) with surrounding granulomatous inflammation, characteristic of tuberculous pleuritis.

of all patients with pulmonary emboli identified on CT pulmonary angiography (CTPA).[73]

Pathophysiology
It is thought that peripheral emboli often cause distal ischemia and pulmonary infarction.[74] Vascular hyperpermeability of capillaries in the pleura or the lung has been hypothesized as a mechanism of pleural fluid accumulation.[75] However, the location of the clots on CTPA and the number of arteries involved do not predict the development of pleural effusions.[73]

Management
Thoracentesis is not routinely indicated because most of these effusions are small and patients are receiving anticoagulants. The effusion is usually an exudate, and pleural fluid shows abundant erythrocytes and polymorphonuclear leukocytes. In one-fifth of patients, pleural fluid eosinophils (more than 10% of total leukocyte count) may be present.[76] Effusion related to pulmonary emboli are usually self-limiting and do not require any specific management. The pleural fluid is often bloody and does not necessarily represent hemorrhage or deter initiation of anticoagulant therapy.[77]

Moderate to large pleural effusions are uncommon after pulmonary emboli and warrant further evaluation to rule out other causes. More importantly, pulmonary embolism should be considered in all patients with an undiagnosed pleural effusion.

Recommended further reading: Findik.[77]

Drug-Induced Pleural Effusion

Numerous drugs have been reported to cause pleural disease with or without concomitant lung parenchymal disease (**Box 1**). Most cases describe an association but not necessarily a causal effect. Drug-induced pleural disease is uncommon, unlike drug-induced lung parenchymal disease.[78] Many drugs (most commonly procainamide, hydralazine and isoniazid) may cause a lupuslike illness, with associated pleuropulmonary manifestations.[79]

Pathophysiology
A hypersensitivity reaction or a direct toxic or inflammatory effect has been postulated.[80]

Clinical presentation
Patents may be asymptomatic, or present with symptoms of acute pleuritis or dyspnea of

---

Box 1
Examples of drugs that can induce pleural effusions

Cardiac Drugs

β-Blockers (practolol, oxyprenolol)

Amiodarone

Minoxidil

Ergoline drugs

Methysergide

Bromocriptine

Ergotamine, dihydroergotamine

Cabergolide

Chemotherapeutic drugs

Bleomycin, mitomycin

Procarbazine

Methotrexate, cyclophosphamide

Docetaxel

Imatinib, desatinib

All-trans retinoic acid, isotretinoin

Immunomodulating drugs

Interferons

Granulocyte-colony stimulating growth factor, intravenous immunoglobulin

Drugs causing lupus pleuritis

Procainamide, hydralazine, isoniazid

Others

Nitrofurantoin, clozapine, valproic acid

Data from Huggins JT, Sahn SA. Drug-induced pleural disease. Clin Chest Med 2004;25:141–53.

without a detailed drug history and high index of suspicion.

Presence of pleural fluid eosinophilia (defined as >10% of nucleated cells), although not specific, is suggestive of drug-induced effusion. Peripheral blood eosinophilia may be present. However, the absence of pleural fluid or blood eosinophilia does not exclude the diagnosis. Most common drugs causing eosinophilic pleural effusion are valproic acid, propylthiouric acid, nitrofurantoin, and bromocryptine.[78]

The pleural fluid in drug-induced lupus is an exudate characterized by normal pH and glucose, increased antinuclear antibodies (ANA) and presence of lupus erythematosus (LE) cells. Increased pleural fluid ANA and LE cells can also be seen in effusions from LE.[79]

Management
Patients may be subjected to an extensive evaluation if drug-induced effusion is not suspected initially. Any drug should be considered as a potential cause, and discontinuation of drugs with or without steroid therapy may be considered if common causes are excluded after an initial evaluation.

For further reading; refer to Huggins and Sahn.[78]

Connective Tissue Diseases

The pleura is variably affected by systemic autoimmune diseases, either in isolation or as part of the systemic involvement. Although seen in association with almost all autoimmune diseases, pleural effusion is most commonly associated with rheumatoid arthritis, systemic LE (SLE), and mixed connective tissue disease, and rarely, systemic sclerosis and polymyositis-dermatomyositis.

Rheumatoid arthritis
Up to 20% of patients with rheumatoid arthritis (RA) may develop symptoms of pleurisy, although not all have radiological evidence of an effusion.[81] RA pleuritis is more common in men, in those with chronic active articular disease and rheumatoid nodules, and in patients with a high RA titer.[82,83] RA is also a risk factor for pseudochylothorax.

Pathophysiology Rupture of rheumatoid nodules into the pleural cavity and subsequent granulomatous inflammation of the pleura is believed to be the cause. The pleural fluid is an exudate characterized by high levels of LDH and low glucose and pH levels caused by ongoing inflammation in the pleural cavity. Rheumatoid nodules, when seen occasionally, are diagnostic, but more often the histologic findings are nonspecific.[81]

thickening is common, although not inev The fluid is characterized by cholesterol and high cholesterol levels.

Clinical presentation The effusion is usua to moderate in size and may be bilateral 25% cases. It may be transient, recur chronic and may be associated with lung chymal abnormalities such as interstitial or rheumatoid nodules. More than half the have subcutaneous nodules. Empyema o mothorax has been reported but is rare.[81]

Management Most RA effusions are asy atic and require no specific treatment. Re to steroids in chronic cases is variable; rec may occur despite treatment. Most cases over 3 to 4 months, but persistent effus affect ~20% of patients. Management of chylothorax is described elsewhere.[85]

SLE
Pleural effusions may be seen in up to patients with SLE, although some effusio be secondary to other manifestations such as heart failure, infection, or pulmon bolism.[86] Many patients may also develop chest pain without an effusion.

Pathophysiology An autoimmune pleu postulated to drive fluid formation.

Clinical presentation Lupus pleuritis is ofte ciated with pleuritic chest pain, fever, an nea.[79] Systemic SLE involvement st pericarditis and lupus pneumonitis may be (**Fig. 5**). Lupus effusions are generally sm may be bilateral. The fluid is usually an e with abundance of neutrophils, although

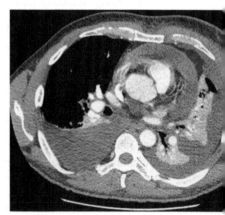

Fig. 5. CT scan showing pericardial and pleural effusions suggestive of pleuroperica a young man, consistent with autoimmune d

effusions may be predominantly lymphocytic. There are no pathognomonic features for SLE effusions. Reduced pleural fluid complement levels, presence of LE cells, increased pleural fluid ANA titers, and pleural fluid/serum ANA ratios greater than 1 are nonspecific findings and in isolation cannot be considered diagnostic.[87]

Management Most small, asymptomatic effusions resolve spontaneously, although corticosteroids and additional immunosuppressive agents may be required for refractory effusions.[88] Pleurodesis may be considered in recurrent effusions.[89]

Postsurgical Pleural Effusions

Pleural effusions are common after surgery. We highlight some of the common and important pleural effusions associated with surgical interventions.

Postcardiac Injury (Dressler's) Syndrome

Pleural effusion can develop after myocardial or pericardial injury of different causes, including myocardial infarction, cardiac surgery, blunt chest trauma, pacemaker implantation, and angioplasty. Postcardiac injury syndrome (PCIS) is characterized by fever, pleuropericarditis, and parenchymal pulmonary infiltrates in the weeks after trauma to the pericardium or myocardium.[90] PCIS is probably immunologically mediated. Myocardial injury may release specific antigens that induce the production of antimyocardial antibodies produced by autosensitization.[91]

Clinical presentation
Chest pain and fever in a patient after myocardial infarction or cardiac surgery is the typical presentation.[91] A pericardial friction rub is present in almost all patients. Peripheral leukocytosis and increased inflammatory markers are common. Chest radiograph usually reveals pulmonary infiltrates. The pleural fluid is usually an exudate and bloody in up to 30% of patients.[92]

Diagnosis is made by exclusion, especially of other diseases that can produce similar symptoms, particularly pleural effusions from postcoronary artery bypass graft (CABG) surgery, CHF, pulmonary embolism, and parapneumonic effusions.[93]

Management
The clinical course is benign and self-limiting. Treatments with nonsteroidal antiinflammatory agents or corticosteroids are usually effective.[94,95] The prognosis of the patient is not altered by development of a pleural effusion.

Post-CABG Surgery Pleural Effusions

Most (~90%) post-CABG patients develop a pleural effusion, which is usually left-sided, small, and self-limiting.[96] However, in 10% of patients, a moderate-sized to large pleural effusion can persist even after 30 days after surgery.[97]

Clinical presentation
Many post-CABG effusions are asymptomatic. Dyspnea can occur, but, unlike PCIS, fever or pain is uncommon. Diagnosis involves exclusion of CHF, pulmonary embolus, infection, chylothorax, and other causes of lymphocyte-rich effusions.[91]

The early, small effusions are probably related to the trauma of surgery and postoperative bleeding. They are usually bloody, with a high red blood cell and eosinophil count and LDH level.[91] The effusions that persist more than 30 days after CABG are predominantly lymphocytic exudates with relatively lower LDH levels.[98] Pleural biopsies often reveal intense lymphocytic pleuritis and, with time, progressive fibrosis. Marked pleural thickening has been reported.[99]

Management
Indications for diagnostic pleural aspiration include if there are symptoms of chest pain or fever, or in the case of a large effusion, if there is dyspnea. Most effusions resolve over time, rarely requiring more than one therapeutic thoracentesis.[97] If the effusion recurs and requires repeated aspirations, a search for alternative causes is recommended before considering pleurodesis. Corticosteroids may help but their role has not been formally defined.

Hemothorax

Hemothorax is, by definition, pleural fluid with a hematocrit level greater than 50% of the blood hematocrit.[100] It is important to distinguish a hemothorax from bloody (hemorrhagic) pleural effusions, because of the different causes. Pleural effusions with a hematocrit level greater than 5% may appear bloody and are often mistaken as a hemothorax, unless the hematocrit is measured.

Pathophysiology
Hemothorax usually signals a more blatant compromise of the vascular wall. The involved vessel could either be a normal vessel undergoing an abnormal stress or an abnormal vessel rupturing without precipitating factors. Bloody (hemorrhagic) effusion can arise from a broad range of causes, including malignancies, TB, uremia, and vascular diseases (eg, pulmonary infarction).

Hemothorax is broadly divided into traumatic, iatrogenic, and spontaneous subtypes (**Table 4**).

Table 4
Examples of common causes of hemothorax

Spontaneous Causes	Traumatic Causes	Iatrogenic Causes
Pneumothorax	Open or penetrating chest	Pleural procedures
Coagulopathy	trauma	Thoracentesis
Congenital: hemophilia	Closed chest trauma	Pleural biopsy
Acquired: anticoagulant		Chest tube insertion
therapy		Intrapleural fibrinolytics
Vascular		Cardiac or thoracic surgery
Arteriovenous malformations		Central venous line insertion
Aortic aneurysms or rupture		
Pulmonary embolism		
Neoplasia		
Lung cancer		
Mesothelioma		
Other metastatic malignancies		
Miscellaneous		
Pulmonary sequestration		
Endometriosis		

Data from Ali HA, Lippmann M, Mundathaje U, et al. Spontaneous hemothorax: a comprehensive review. Chest 2008;134(5):1056–65; and Light RW, Lee YC. Pneumothorax, chylothorax, hemothorax and fibrothorax. In: Mason R, Broaddus VC, Martin TR, et al, editors. Murray & Nadel's textbook of respiratory diseases. 5th edition. Philadelphia: Saunders Elsevier; 2010. p. 1764–91.

Traumatic hemothorax often results from open or closed chest trauma, including interventional (eg, pleural) procedures (**Fig. 6**). Spontaneous hemothorax can occur and complicates 3% to 7% of spontaneous pneumothoraces.[101,102] Pleural malignancy can bleed into the pleural cavity. Patients with pulmonary emboli/infarct treated with anticoagulation therapy are also at risk.[103] Catamenial hemothorax is a rare but documented cause.

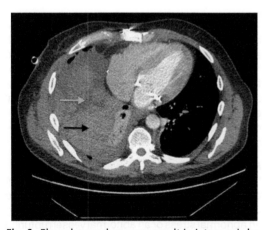

Fig. 6. Pleural procedures may result in iatrogenic hemothorax. CT scan in a patient after pleural procedure showing a heterogeneous abnormality within the pleural space. Pleural fluid appears less dense (*gray arrow*) and blood has a relatively higher density (*black arrow*). Subsequent chest tube drainage of frank blood confirmed hemothorax.

Management

Hemothorax should be suspected in any patient who develops a pleural effusion after suffering a penetrating or nonpenetrating trauma to the chest. A hemothorax may be minute or absent on an initial chest radiograph. A traumatic hemothorax should be promptly drained with a large-bore tube to reduce risk of subsequent empyema and fibrothorax and to quantify the rate of blood loss. Bleeding at a rate of more than 200 mL/h is usually considered an indication for surgical intervention[104] or transcatheter arterial embolization of the bleeding intercostal artery.[105]

Prophylactic antibiotics significantly reduced pleural infections after chest trauma needing tube thoracostomy in some studies,[106,107] but not in others.[108]

Chylothorax

Presence of chyle in the pleural space defines a chylothorax. Chyle is lymph fluid rich in chylomicrons and triglyceride. Chylothorax should be differentiated from pseudochylothorax; both appear milky. A pseudochylothorax is characterized by the presence of cholesterol or lecithin-globulin complexes but lacks chylomicrons.

Pathophysiology

Chyle passes from the intestinal lymphatics via the cisterna chyli into the thoracic duct to drain into the venous system. Chylothorax develops when

the course of the thoracic duct. The duct is susceptible to injury during surgical procedures (especially those involving the posterior mediastinum), because its course is often anomalous and variations are common. The side of the chylothorax depends on the level of the anatomic disruption because the thoracic duct crosses over from the right side of the thorax to the left at the level of T3-T4 vertebra.[85]

Between 1.5 and 2.5 L of chyle empties into the venous system daily. Chyle leak may result in severe depletion of volume, nutrition, electrolytes, and lymphocytes; hence, its early recognition and prompt treatment are necessary.

Disruption of the thoracic duct from trauma (including surgery) and nontraumatic causes can lead to chylothoraces (**Table 5**). Numerous case reports have linked chylothorax with various (including trivial) trauma. The incidence after thoracic surgery is around 0.5%.[85] Practically any surgical procedures involving the heart, mediastinum, or neck, including insertion of catheters or pacemakers,[109] have been associated with chylothoraces.

commonest nontraumatic cause of chylothorax, presumably because of compression/obstruction of the duct by tumor or mediastinal lymphadenopathy. Destruction of the lymphatics after radiation therapy is another known cause.[110]

Clinical manifestation

Dyspnea is the usual presenting symptom and its severity depends on the size and rapidity of chyle accumulation. Traumatic effusions tend to develop more rapidly. Chest pain and fever are uncommon.

Chylothorax often has a distinctive milky appearance, which can be absent if the patient is starved. Presence of chylomicrons in the pleural fluid defines chylothorax. Alternatively, an increased pleural fluid triglyceride level is often used as a surrogate diagnostic criterion.[111] Presence of cholesterol crystals or increased pleural fluid cholesterol level suggests a pseudochylothorax instead.

Management

Chylothorax should be suspected in pleural effusions after trauma or thoracic surgery. In

---

Table 5
Causes of chylothorax

Medical Causes	Traumatic Causes
Neoplasms	Iatrogenic
Lymphoma	Thoracic surgery
Bronchogenic carcinoma	(eg, posterior mediastinal surgery)
Lymphoproliferative disorders	Surgery of head and neck
Benign tumors	(eg, radical neck dissection)
Retrosternal goiter	Celiac plexus block
Diseases affecting lymphatic drainage	Subclavian catheter insertion
Infections	Pacemaker insertion
TB	Noniatrogenic trauma
Filariasis	Penetrating or crush trauma
Congenital	Forceful cough or vomiting
Yellow nail syndrome	Childbirth
Lymphangioleiomyomatosis	
Intestinal lymphatic dysplasia	
Primary lymphatic dysplasia	
Congenital pulmonary lymphangiectasis	
Others causes	
Amyloidosis	
Sarcoidosis	
Postirradiation	
Hypothyroidism	
Cirrhosis of liver	
Thrombosis of superior vena cava	
or central veins	

Data from Light RW, Lee YC. Pneumothorax, chylothorax, hemothorax and fibrothorax. In: Mason R, Broaddus VC, Martin TR, et al, editors. Murray & Nadel's textbook of respiratory diseases. 5th edition. Philadelphia: Saunders Elsevier; 2010. p. 1764–91.

astinal lymphadenopathy (especially from lymphoma) and tumors.

Management of chylothorax is complex and includes treating the underlying cause, maintaining nutritional status by reducing chyle loss, and relieving symptoms. Trauma to the thoracic duct usually heals with time. Reducing the chyle flow may aid healing. Chyle flow can be reduced by using total parenteral nutrition or medium-chain triglyceride. Patients with mediastinal tumors/lymphadenopathy may respond to chemoirradiation to reduce lymphatic obstruction and chyle leak.

Prolonged leak may require surgical repair or ligation of the thoracic duct. Obliteration of the duct by interventional radiological means has also been shown to be successful. Pleurodesis can be considered. Thoracentesis is useful in improving symptoms, but frequent drainage of chylothorax can lead to malnutrition and immunodeficiency. Nonetheless, IPC has been used in selected patients with cancer-related chylothorax.[112]

Benign Asbestos Pleural Effusion

Asbestos exposure may lead to mesothelioma as well as a range of benign pleural diseases, including pleural plaques, diffuse pleural thickening, rolled atelectasis, and benign asbestos pleural effusion (BAPE). BAPE has a median latency of 16 years between first exposure and effusion development.[113] BAPE is a risk factor for the subsequent development of diffuse pleural thickening.[113]

Clinical presentation

BAPE is a diagnosis by exclusion, especially for mesothelioma. The effusion is usually small, unilateral, an exudate, and often hemorrhagic.[114,115] Patients may be asymptomatic.[114] Fever is uncommon, but other inflammatory markers may be raised. Biopsies usually show pleural fibrosis or inflammatory mesothelial and fibroblastic proliferation. The effusion usually resolves spontaneously over a few months, but can recur occasionally.[115] Definitive procedures such as pleurodesis are seldom needed. Follow-up to exclude mesothelioma is warranted (**Fig. 7**).[116]

For further reading; refer to Musk and De Klerk.[116]

SUMMARY

Benign pleural effusions are common and of varied causes, often causing diagnostic and management challenges. A systematic approach embracing

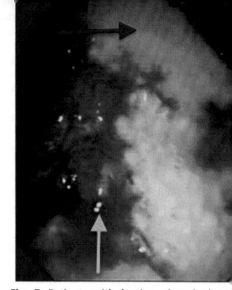

Fig. 7. Patients with benign pleural plaqu exposure to asbestos may subsequently malignant mesothelioma. Pleuroscopy showin sive benign pleural plaques (*black arrow*). Adj it are pleural nodules (*gray arrow*) caused b thelioma, which was confirmed by biopsy.

clinical history, appropriate imaging, and fluid/tissue sampling is necessary to estal accurate diagnosis.

REFERENCES

1. Light RW. Pleural diseases. 4th edition. E (MD): Williams & Wilkins; 1995.
2. Marel M, Zrustova M, Stasny B, et al. The ir of pleural effusion in a well-defined regior miologic study in central Bohemia. Che 104:1486–9.
3. Light RW, Lee YCG, editors. Textbook o diseases. 2nd edition. London: Hodder 2008.
4. Noppen M, De Waele M, Li R, et al. Volu cellular content of normal pleural fluid in examined by pleural lavage. Am J Re Care Med 2000;162:1023–6.
5. English JC, Leslie KO. Pathology of the ple Chest Med 2006;27:157–80.
6. Broaddus VC, Light RW. What is the (pleural transudates and exudates? Che 102:658–9.
7. Light RW, Macgregor MI, Luchsinger PC, et a effusions: the diagnostic separation of trar and exudates. Ann Intern Med 1972;77:507
8. Heffner JE, Brown LK, Barbieri CA. Di value of tests that discriminate between e

and transducive pleural effusions. Primary Study Investigators. Chest 1997;111:970–80.

9. Light RW. Diagnostic principles in pleural disease. Eur Respir J 1997;10:476–81.

10. Lee YC, Davies RJ, Light RW. Diagnosing pleural effusion: moving beyond transudate-exudate separation. Chest 2007;131:942–3.

11. Hooper C, Lee YC, Maskell N, et al. Investigation of a unilateral pleural effusion in adults: British Thoracic Society Pleural Disease Guideline 2010. Thorax 2010;65(Suppl 2):ii4–17.

12. Light RW. Pleural effusions. Med Clin North Am 2011;95:1055–70.

13. Wiener-Kronish JP, Matthay MA, Callen PW, et al. Relationship of pleural effusions to pulmonary hemodynamics in patients with congestive heart failure. Am Rev Respir Dis 1985;132:1253–6.

14. Tang KJ, Robbins IM, Light RW. Incidence of pleural effusions in idiopathic and familial pulmonary arterial hypertension patients. Chest 2009;136: 688–93.

15. Edwards JE, Race GA, Scheifley CH. Hydrothorax in congestive heart failure. Am J Med 1957;22:83–9.

16. Natanzon A, Kronzon I. Pericardial and pleural effusions in congestive heart failure–anatomical, pathophysiologic, and clinical considerations. Am J Med Sci 2009;338:211–6.

17. Romero-Candeira S, Fernandez C, Martin C, et al. Influence of diuretics on the concentration of proteins and other components of pleural transudates in patients with heart failure. Am J Med 2001;110:681–6.

18. Porcel JM, Martinez-Alonso M, Cao G, et al. Biomarkers of heart failure in pleural fluid. Chest 2009;136:671–7.

19. Glazer M, Berkman N, Lafair JS, et al. Successful talc slurry pleurodesis in patients with nonmalignant pleural effusion. Chest 2000;117:1404–9.

20. Weiss JM, Spodick DH. Association of left pleural effusion with pericardial disease. N Engl J Med 1983;308:696–7.

21. Giacobbe A, Facciorusso D, Barbano F, et al. Hepatic hydrothorax. Diagnosis and management. Clin Nucl Med 1996;21:56–60.

22. Kinasewitz GT. Transudative effusions. Eur Respir J 1997;10:714–8.

23. Roussos A, Philippou N, Mantzaris GJ, et al. Hepatic hydrothorax: pathophysiology diagnosis and management. J Gastroenterol Hepatol 2007; 22:1388–93.

24. Lieberman FL, Hidemura R, Peters RL, et al. Pathogenesis and treatment of hydrothorax complicating cirrhosis with ascites. Ann Intern Med 1966;64:341–51.

25. Alberts WM, Salem AJ, Solomon DA, et al. Hepatic hydrothorax. Cause and management. Arch Intern Med 1991;151:2383–8.

26. Ackerman Z, Reynolds TB. Evaluation of pleural fluid in patients with cirrhosis. J Clin Gastroenterol 1997;25:619–22.

27. Xiol X, Castellote J, Cortes-Beut R, et al. Usefulness and complications of thoracentesis in cirrhotic patients. Am J Med 2001;111:67–9.

28. Xiol X, Castellvi JM, Guardiola J, et al. Spontaneous bacterial empyema in cirrhotic patients: a prospective study. Hepatology 1996;23:719–23.

29. Malagari K, Nikita A, Alexopoulou E, et al. Cirrhosis-related intrathoracic disease. Imaging features in 1038 patients. Hepatogastroenterology 2005;52:558–62.

30. Romero S, Martin C, Hernandez L, et al. Chylothorax in cirrhosis of the liver: analysis of its frequency and clinical characteristics. Chest 1998;114:154–9.

31. Xiol X, Tremosa G, Castellote J, et al. Liver transplantation in patients with hepatic hydrothorax. Transpl Int 2005;18:672–5.

32. Kinasewitz GT, Keddissi JI. Hepatic hydrothorax. Curr Opin Pulm Med 2003;9:261–5.

33. Spencer EB, Cohen DT, Darcy MD. Safety and efficacy of transjugular intrahepatic portosystemic shunt creation for the treatment of hepatic hydrothorax. J Vasc Interv Radiol 2002;13:385–90.

34. Wongcharatrawee S, Garcia-Tsao G. Clinical management of ascites and its complications. Clin Liver Dis 2001;5:833–50.

35. Takahashi K, Chin K, Sumi K, et al. Resistant hepatic hydrothorax: a successful case with treatment by nCPAP. Respir Med 2005;99:262–4.

36. Cerfolio RJ, Bryant AS. Efficacy of video-assisted thoracoscopic surgery with talc pleurodesis for porous diaphragm syndrome in patients with refractory hepatic hydrothorax. Ann Thorac Surg 2006;82:457–9.

37. Mercky P, Sakr L, Heyries L, et al. Use of a tunnelled pleural catheter for the management of refractory hepatic hydrothorax: a new therapeutic option. Respiration 2010;80:348–52.

38. Niederman MS, Mandell LA, Anzueto A, et al. Guidelines for the management of adults with community-acquired pneumonia. Diagnosis, assessment of severity, antimicrobial therapy, and prevention. Am J Respir Crit Care Med 2001;163: 1730–54.

39. Wrightson JM, Davies HE, Lee YC. Pleural effusion, empyema and pneumothorax. In: Spiro SG, Agusti A, Silvestri G, editors. Clinical respiratory medicine. 4th edition. Philadelphia: Elsevier; 2012. p. 69.1–69.19.

40. Hasley PB, Albaum MN, Li YH, et al. Do pulmonary radiographic findings at presentation predict mortality in patients with community-acquired pneumonia? Arch Intern Med 1996;156:2206–12.

41. Maskell NA, Davies CW, Nunn AJ, et al. U.K. controlled trial of intrapleural streptokinase for pleural infection. N Engl J Med 2005;352:865–74.

42. Maskell NA, Batt S, Hedley EL, et al. The bacteriology of pleural infection by genetic and standard methods and its mortality significance. Am J Respir Crit Care Med 2006;174:817–23.

43. Chalmers JD, Singanayagam A, Murray MP, et al. Risk factors for complicated parapneumonic effusion and empyema on presentation to hospital with community-acquired pneumonia. Thorax 2009;64:592–7.

44. Falguera M, Carratala J, Bielsa S, et al. Predictive factors, microbiology and outcome of patients with parapneumonic effusion. Eur Respir J 2011; 38:1173–9.

45. Chu MW, Dewar LR, Burgess JJ, et al. Empyema thoracis: lack of awareness results in a prolonged clinical course. Can J Surg 2001;44:284–8.

46. LeMense GP, Strange C, Sahn SA. Empyema thoracis. Therapeutic management and outcome. Chest 1995;107:1532–7.

47. Shankar S, Gulati M, Kang M, et al. Image-guided percutaneous drainage of thoracic empyema: can sonography predict the outcome? Eur Radiol 2000;10:495–9.

48. Rahman NM, Maskell NA, Davies CW, et al. The relationship between chest tube size and clinical outcome in pleural infection. Chest 2010;137: 536–43.

49. Rahman NM, Maskell NA, West A, et al. Intrapleural use of tissue plasminogen activator and DNase in pleural infection. N Engl J Med 2011;365:518–26.

50. Davies HE, Davies RJ, Davies CW, et al. Management of pleural infection in adults: British Thoracic Society Pleural Disease Guideline 2010. Thorax 2010;65(Suppl 2):ii41–53.

51. Cassina PC, Hauser M, Hillejan L, et al. Video-assisted thoracoscopy in the treatment of pleural empyema: stage-based management and outcome. J Thorac Cardiovasc Surg 1999;117: 234–8.

52. St Peter SD, Tsao K, Spilde TL, et al. Thoracoscopic decortication vs tube thoracostomy with fibrinolysis for empyema in children: a prospective, randomized trial. J Pediatr Surg 2009;44:106–11 [discussion: 11].

53. Wait MA, Sharma S, Hohn J, et al. A randomized trial of empyema therapy. Chest 1997;111: 1548–51.

54. Bilgin M, Akcali Y, Oguzkaya F. Benefits of early aggressive management of empyema thoracis. ANZ J Surg 2006;76:120–2.

55. Kurt BA, Winterhalter KM, Connors RH, et al. Therapy of parapneumonic effusions in children: video-assisted thoracoscopic surgery versus conventional thoracostomy drainage. Pediatrics 2006;118:e547–53.

56. Sonnappa S, Cohen G, Owens CM, et al. Comparison of urokinase and video-assisted thoracoscopic surgery for treatment of childhood empyema. Am J Respir Crit Care Med 2006;174: 221–7.

57. Diacon AH, Theron J, Schuurmans MM, et al. Intrapleural streptokinase for empyema and complicated parapneumonic effusions. Am J Respir Crit Care Med 2004;170:49–53.

58. Mlika-Cabanne N, Brauner M, Kamanfu G, et al. Radiographic abnormalities in tuberculosis and risk of coexisting human immunodeficiency virus infection. Methods and preliminary results from Bujumbura, Burundi. Am J Respir Crit Care Med 1995;152:794–9.

59. Baumann MH, Nolan R, Petrini M, et al. Pleural tuberculosis in the United States: incidence and drug resistance. Chest 2007;131:1125–32.

60. Pozniak AL, MacLeod GA, Ndlovu D, et al. Clinical and chest radiographic features of tuberculosis associated with human immunodeficiency virus in Zimbabwe. Am J Respir Crit Care Med 1995;152: 1558–61.

61. Moudgil H, Sridhar G, Leitch AG. Reactivation disease: the commonest form of tuberculous pleural effusion in Edinburgh, 1980-1991. Respir Med 1994;88:301–4.

62. Berger HW, Mejia E. Tuberculous pleurisy. Chest 1973;63:88–92.

63. Escudero Bueno C, Garcia Clemente M, Cuesta Castro B, et al. Cytologic and bacteriologic analysis of fluid and pleural biopsy specimens with Cope's needle. Study of 414 patients. Arch Intern Med 1990;150:1190–4.

64. Valdes L, Alvarez D, San Jose E, et al. Tuberculous pleurisy: a study of 254 patients. Arch Intern Med 1998;158:2017–21.

65. Kim HJ, Lee HJ, Kwon SY, et al. The prevalence of pulmonary parenchymal tuberculosis in patients with tuberculous pleuritis. Chest 2006;129:1253–8.

66. Conde MB, Loivos AC, Rezende VM, et al. Yield of sputum induction in the diagnosis of pleural tuberculosis. Am J Respir Crit Care Med 2003; 167:723–5.

67. Diacon AH, Van de Wal BW, Wyser C, et al. Diagnostic tools in tuberculous pleurisy: a direct comparative study. Eur Respir J 2003;22:589–91.

68. Liang QL, Shi HZ, Wang K, et al. Diagnostic accuracy of adenosine deaminase in tuberculous pleurisy: a meta-analysis. Respir Med 2008;102: 744–54.

69. Roper WH, Waring JJ. Primary serofibrinous pleural effusion in military personnel. Am Rev Tuberc 1955; 71:616–34.

70. Light RW. Update on tuberculous pleural effusion. Respirology 2010;15:451–8.

71. Al-Majed SA. Study of paradoxical response to chemotherapy in tuberculous pleural effusion. Respir Med 1996;90:211–4.

72. Barbas CS, Cukier A, de Varvalho CR, et al. The relationship between pleural fluid findings and the development of pleural thickening in patients with pleural tuberculosis. Chest 1991;100:1264–7.

73. Yap E, Anderson G, Donald J, et al. Pleural effusion in patients with pulmonary embolism. Respirology 2008;13:832–6.

74. Light RW. Pleural effusion due to pulmonary emboli. Curr Opin Pulm Med 2001;7:198–201.

75. Porcel JM, Madronero AB, Pardina M, et al. Analysis of pleural effusions in acute pulmonary embolism: radiological and pleural fluid data from 230 patients. Respirology 2007;12:234–9.

76. Romero Candeira S, Hernandez Blasco L, Soler MJ, et al. Biochemical and cytologic characteristics of pleural effusions secondary to pulmonary embolism. Chest 2002;121:465–9.

77. Findik S. Pleural effusion in pulmonary embolism. Curr Opin Pulm Med 2012;18:347–54.

78. Huggins JT, Sahn SA. Drug-induced pleural disease. Clin Chest Med 2004;25:141–53.

79. Good JT Jr, King TE, Antony VB, et al. Lupus pleuritis. Clinical features and pleural fluid characteristics with special reference to pleural fluid antinuclear antibodies. Chest 1983;84:714–8.

80. Antony VB. Drug-induced pleural disease. Clin Chest Med 1998;19:331–40.

81. Bouros D, Pneumatikos I, Tzouvelekis A. Pleural involvement in systemic autoimmune disorders. Respiration 2008;75:361–71.

82. Highland KB, Heffner JE. Pleural effusion in interstitial lung disease. Curr Opin Pulm Med 2004;10:390–6.

83. Balbir-Gurman A, Yigla M, Nahir AM, et al. Rheumatoid pleural effusion. Semin Arthritis Rheum 2006;35:368–78.

84. Wrightson JM, Stanton AE, Maskell NA, et al. Pseudochylothorax without pleural thickening: time to reconsider pathogenesis? Chest 2009;136:1144–7.

85. Hillerdal G. Effusions from lymphatic disruptions. In: Light RW, Lee YC, editors. Textbook of pleural diseases. London: Hodder Arnold; 2008. p. 393–4.

86. Pines A, Kaplinsky N, Olchovsky D, et al. Pleuropulmonary manifestations of systemic lupus erythematosus: clinical features of its subgroups. Prognostic and therapeutic implications. Chest 1985;88:129–35.

87. Khare V, Baethge B, Lang S, et al. Antinuclear antibodies in pleural fluid. Chest 1994;106:866–71.

88. Brasington RD, Furst DE. Pulmonary disease in systemic lupus erythematosus. Clin Exp Rheumatol 1985;3:269–76.

89. Kaine JL. Refractory massive pleural effusion in systemic lupus erythematosus treated with talc poudrage. Ann Rheum Dis 1985;44:61–4.

90. Dressler W. The post-myocardial-infarction syndrome: a report on forty-four cases. AMA Arch Intern Med 1959;103:28–42.

91. Light RW. Pleural effusions following cardiac injury and coronary artery bypass graft surgery. Semin Respir Crit Care Med 2001;22:657–64.

92. Stelzner TJ, King TE Jr, Antony VB, et al. The pleuropulmonary manifestations of the postcardiac injury syndrome. Chest 1983;84:383–7.

93. King TE Jr, Stelzner TJ, Sahn SA. Cardiac tamponade complicating the postpericardiotomy syndrome. Chest 1983;83:500–3.

94. Gregoratos G. Pericardial involvement in acute myocardial infarction. Cardiol Clin 1990;8:601–8.

95. Heidecker J, Sahn SA. The spectrum of pleural effusions after coronary artery bypass grafting surgery. Clin Chest Med 2006;27:267–83.

96. Vargas FS, Cukier A, Hueb W, et al. Relationship between pleural effusion and pericardial involvement after myocardial revascularization. Chest 1994;105:1748–52.

97. Light RW, Rogers JT, Moyers JP, et al. Prevalence and clinical course of pleural effusions at 30 days after coronary artery and cardiac surgery. Am J Respir Crit Care Med 2002;166:1567–71.

98. Sadikot RT, Rogers JT, Cheng DS, et al. Pleural fluid characteristics of patients with symptomatic pleural effusion after coronary artery bypass graft surgery. Arch Intern Med 2000;160:2665–8.

99. Lee YC, Vaz MA, Ely KA, et al. Symptomatic persistent post-coronary artery bypass graft pleural effusions requiring operative treatment: clinical and histologic features. Chest 2001;119:795–800.

100. Light RW. Pleural diseases. 5th edition. Baltimore (MD): Lippincott Williams & Wilkins; 2007.

101. Hsu NY, Shih CS, Hsu CP, et al. Spontaneous hemopneumothorax revisited: clinical approach and systemic review of the literature. Ann Thorac Surg 2005;80:1859–63.

102. Ali HA, Lippmann M, Mundathaje U, et al. Spontaneous hemothorax: a comprehensive review. Chest 2008;134(5):1056–65.

103. Light RW, Lee YC. Pneumothorax, chylothorax, hemothorax and fibrothorax. In: Mason R, Broaddus VC, Martin TR, et al, editors. Murray & Nadel's textbook of respiratory diseases. 5th edition. Philadelphia: Saunders Elsevier; 2010. p. 1764–91.

104. Carrillo EH, Richardson JD. Thoracoscopy in the management of hemothorax and retained blood after trauma. Curr Opin Pulm Med 1998;4:243–6.

105. Hagiwara A, Yanagawa Y, Kaneko N, et al. Indications for transcatheter arterial embolization in persistent hemothorax caused by blunt trauma. J Trauma 2008;65:589–94.

106. Gonzalez RP, Holevar MR. Role of prophylactic antibiotics for tube thoracostomy in chest trauma. Am Surg 1998;64:617–20 [discussion: 20–1].

107. Brunner RG, Vinsant GO, Alexander RH, et al. The role of antibiotic therapy in the prevention of

empyema in patients with an isolated chest injury (ISS 9-10): a prospective study. J Trauma 1990; 30:1148–53 [discussion: 53–4].

108. Maxwell RA, Campbell DJ, Fabian TC, et al. Use of presumptive antibiotics following tube thoracostomy for traumatic hemopneumothorax in the prevention of empyema and pneumonia–a multi-center trial. J Trauma 2004;57:742–8 [discussion: 8–9].

109. Thomas R, Christopher DJ, Roy A, et al. Chylothorax following innominate vein thrombosis–a rare complication of transvenous pacemaker implantation. Respiration 2007;74:338–40.

110. Talwar A, Lee HJ. A contemporary review of chylothorax. Indian J Chest Dis Allied Sci 2008;50: 343–51.

111. Staats BA, Ellefson RD, Budahn LL, et al. The lipoprotein profile of chylous and nonchylous pleural effusions. Mayo Clin Proc 1980;55:700–4.

112. Jimenez CA, Mhatre AD, Martinez CH, et al. Use of an indwelling pleural catheter for the management of recurrent chylothorax in patients with cancer. Chest 2007;132:1584–90.

113. Cookson WO, De Klerk NH, Musk AW, et al. Benign and malignant pleural effusions in former Wittenoom crocidolite millers and miners. Aust N Z J Med 1985;15:731–7.

114. Epler GR, McLoud TC, Gaensler EA. Prevalence and incidence of benign asbestos pleural effusion in a working population. JAMA 1982;247:617–22.

115. Robinson BW, Musk AW. Benign asbestos pleural effusion: diagnosis and course. Thorax 1981;36: 896–900.

116. Musk AW, De Klerk NH. Asbestos related pleural diseases. In: Light RW, Lee YC, editors. Textbook of pleural diseases. 2nd edition. London: Hodder Arnold; 2008. p. 499–505.

Surgical Management of Malignant Pleural Effusions

Sudish C. Murthy, MD, PhD[a],*, Thomas W. Rice, MD[b]

KEYWORDS

- Thoracentesis • Tunneled pleural catheter • Video-assisted thoracic surgery • Talc poudrage
- Decortication

KEY POINTS

- Thoracentesis helps in diagnosis and end-of-life palliation of malignant pleural effusions (MPE). Other strategies are necessary for palliation of patients with potential "long-term" survival.
- Tunneled pleural catheters (TPCs) provide a simple and effective treatment of MPE, particularly in patients with entrapped lung. Major disadvantages are the existence of an external foreign body and the need for ongoing drainage.
- Video-assisted thoracic surgery (VATS) talc poudrage provides efficacious and durable pleurodesis and palliation of dyspnea. A general anesthetic is required, but this is theoretically a one-event procedure for managing MPE.
- Decortication is practiced to some extent at all diagnostic and therapeutic VATS procedures for MPE. This procedure, particularly at thoracotomy, should be reserved for palliation of malignant mesothelioma.
- Surgical management of MPE requires balancing the patients' wishes, performance status, and prognosis with the ability to obtain full lung expansion and control fluid production. There is no ideal procedure; surgical treatment must be individualized.

Prompt and durable control of symptomatic MPE is of paramount importance because those afflicted have generally entered the terminal phase of their illness, and quality of life becomes the central role of therapy. To this end, several palliative interventions can be considered. The simplest of these is thoracentesis, which should be reserved for patients in whom end of life is rapidly approaching, as evidenced by very poor performance status and severe debility not simply attributable to the mechanical effects of MPE.[1,2] Because recurrence of MPE after thoracentesis approaches 100% within 1 month, other strategies must be considered for patients with greater predicted survival.

More invasive options include temporary chest drain with or without chemical sclerosis, tunneled (indwelling) catheter, medical thorascopy and pleurodesis, VATS and talc poudrage, and rarely, decortication.

PATIENT IDENTIFICATION

Although there are no firm guidelines to direct which patients should be offered more invasive therapies for MPE, there are important data that suggest patient groups that might benefit the least. Prognostic factors for survival after surgical palliation of MPE include leukocytosis, hypoxemia,

---

[a] Department of Thoracic and Cardiovascular Surgery, Heart and Vascular Institute, Cleveland Clinic, 9500 Euclid Avenue/Desk J4–1, Cleveland, OH 44195, USA; [b] Department of Thoracic and Cardiovascular Surgery, Heart and Vascular Institute, Cleveland Clinic Lerner College of Medicine, Cleveland Clinic, 9500 Euclid Avenue/Desk J4–1, Cleveland, OH 44195, USA
* Corresponding author. Department of Thoracic and Cardiovascular Surgery, Cleveland Clinic, 9500 Euclid Avenue/Desk J4-1, Cleveland, OH 44195.
E-mail address: murthys1@ccf.org

Thorac Surg Clin 23 (2013) 43–49
http://dx.doi.org/10.1016/j.thorsurg.2012.10.001

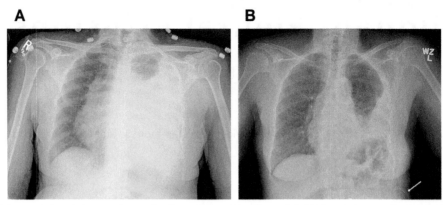

Fig. 1. (*A*) Preprocedural chest radiograph of a patient with a large left MPE, causing mediastinal shift, complicating breast cancer. (*B*) Effective palliation of the patient's shortness of breath was obtained with a TPC (*arrow*) despite failure to obtain complete expansion of the partially entrapped left lung.

and hypoalbuminemia.[3] For patients in whom these factors coexist, survival seems markedly worse than for patients who have none, approaching 6 weeks. Consequently, these patients and others with very poor performance status should be steered away from more morbid invasive treatment options and toward medical therapies.[1]

With rare exceptions, MPE presenting with trapped lung should fall out of the purview of standard surgical palliation. These patients might be difficult to identify unless a prior thoracentesis has demonstrated the syndrome. Lung entrapment is incidentally noted in a surprisingly high number of patients with MPE and is not effectively palliated by surgical intervention.[4] Patients with trapped lung seem best served by less-invasive treatments (**Fig. 1**).[4–6]

TUNNELED PLEURAL CATHETERS

Introduction of the (indwelling) TPC has provided a simple and effective treatment of MPE (**Fig. 2**). However, there is no consensus regarding the optimal treatment of symptomatic MPE for reasonably fit patients without significant lung entrapment. Published debates on the subject exist, and cogent arguments can be made in support of either TPC or VATS talc poudrage.[7,8] Data on both sides of the debate are surprisingly robust, although a direct randomized comparison between the 2 approaches has not yet been completed. A recent randomized study favors TPC over bedside-delivered talc slurry (TS),[9] but equivalence between TS and VATS poudrage has never been truly established. In fact, the preponderance of data favors the contrary, that is, that the 2 are not equivalent and that VATS poudrage is more efficacious.[10–12] Moreover, TS can be associated with more procedural pain than VATS.[11]

The efficacy of TPC for MPE, compared with doxycycline pleurodesis, was established several years ago.[13] Despite doxycycline being an inferior sclerosant to talc,[10] the utility of TPC for MPE is undeniable. Proponents cite that TPC offers rapid palliation of dyspnea with limited hospital stay and excellent patient satisfaction.[4,13,14] Immediate

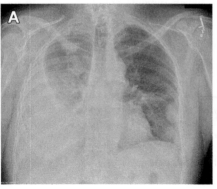
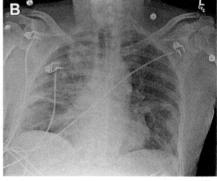

Fig. 2. (*A*) Preprocedural chest radiograph of a patient with a right MPE complicating non–small cell lung cancer. (*B*) Immediate postprocedure chest radiograph after placement of a TPC.

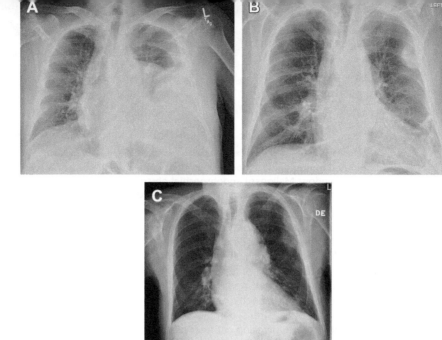

Fig. 3. (*A*) Preprocedural chest radiograph of a patient with a symptomatic recurrent left MPE after thoracentesis. He was receiving a kinase inhibitor (axitinib) for diffusely metastatic renal cell cancer to bone, brain, and pleura. (*B*) Chest radiograph 2 months after removal of TPC. (*C*) Chest radiograph 1 month after TPC removal demonstrates successful pleurodesis and excellent control of left pleural space.

procedure-related costs (often compared with VATS) seem lower, although late costs are generally underappreciated.[4] Finally, the ease of placement has allowed for rapid dissemination of TPC, which can be placed anywhere from the operating room to the radiology suite.[15]

There are, however, several important drawbacks associated with TPCs. Catheter dysfunction is not uncommon, and intermittent thrombolysis

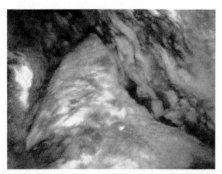

Fig. 4. View of the right pleural space at VATS after effective application of talc by aerosol spray. Successful pleurodesis requires exposure of the entire pleural surface to talc. This exposure is accomplished by complete drainage of all pleural fluid and sequential exposure of segments of the pleura to the aerosol. Settling of the aerosolized talc onto the pleural surface is preferred to direct application to the surface. This process requires multiple applications of talc, meticulous exposure of all pleura surfaces, repeated visual assessment, and above all, patience.

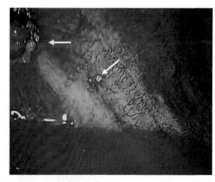

Fig. 5. View of the left pleural space at diagnostic VATS. Draining pleural fluid, which was cytologically negative at thoracentesis, exposed unsuspected pleural metastases (*arrows*). Biopsy and frozen section analysis revealed metastatic adenocarcinoma. Informed consent had been obtained because this potential diagnosis had been considered, and thus it was possible to perform talc poudrage under the same anesthesia.

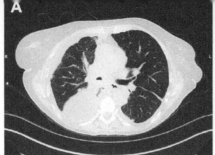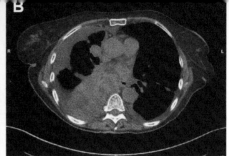

Fig. 6. Computed tomographic images of a patient with stage IV breast cancer and MPE. (*A*) Lung wind (*B*) mediastinal window. Malignant endobronchial obstruction of the right lower lobe prevented reexpa the involved right lung. Bronchoscopy was critical in avoiding fruitless VATS and attempted talc pleuro

might be required to maintain long-term catheter patency.[4–6,15] Catheter tract seeding has been reported in 7% of patients and can ultimately lead to additional interventions.[16] Also, up to 10% of TPCs fracture during removal, and two-thirds of these cases result in permanently retained catheter fragments.[17] The disastrous complication of empyema secondary to indwelling catheter placement or use negates any palliation gained from this approach and elevates the complexity of management manyfold.

Perhaps the most glaring deficiency of TPC use for MPE is that spontaneous pleurodesis does not occur in most patients.[4,13–15,18] Randomized data suggest that the pleurodesis rate from TPC is almost 20% less than that of bedside pleurodesis and that lung expansion is worse.[9] This observation presumably translates into long-term TPC use for MPE control and perhaps late patient dissatisfaction, which is unreported in most studies. Interestingly, successful pleurodesis has been postulated to account for improved survival for patients with MPE (**Fig. 3**),[19,20] which would lead to the argument that both palliation of

dyspnea and successful pleurodesis are in metrics on which to base treatment strateg failure of TPCs in this regard has been appr by some, as concomitant TPC placement instillation with medical thorascopy has b tempted.[21] This approach has unfortunate accompanied by a 7% catheter failure/er rate. Paradoxically, when pleurodesis possible, as seen with entrapped lu tunneled catheter has proved to be highly e and better than bedside talc pleuroc managing this complication of MPE.[9]

VATS TALC PLEURODESIS

Surgical management of MPE typically beg ends with VATS talc poudrage (**Fig. 4**). Th duction of video thoracoscopy several ye dramatically reduced morbidity (associat more invasive operations) and expedited r of patients undergoing surgical pleurode efficacy of the procedure has been confir systematic data reviews and palliation of c and pleurodesis rates approaching 90%,[1

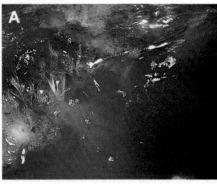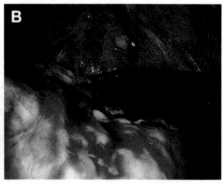

Fig. 7. (*A*) The initial view at VATS of a multiloculated MPE. This should not discourage the surgeon from e rupturing, debriding, and evacuating all loculations. (*B*) View at VATS after meticulously breaking down lations and before complete evacuation of pleural fluid in preparation for talc pleurodesis.

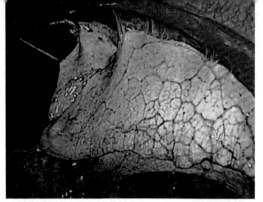

Fig. 8. View at VATS of filmy adhesions complicating failed chemical pleurodesis for MPE. Adhesiolysis is frequently required and easily performed to improve talc pleurodesis.

the durability of the procedure has long since been documented. Guidelines highlighting the central role of VATS pleurodesis for MPE have been established.[22]

In the clinical situation in which VATS is prescribed to determine the cause of pleural effusions, the possibility of a malignant effusion should always be considered and discussed with the patient before surgery. Informed consent includes

Depending on the operative findings at VATS and frozen section pathologic review of the biopsy material, it may be in the patient's best interest to palliate the malignant effusion at the time of diagnosis and avoid further anesthetics and additional procedures (**Fig. 5**).

Bronchoscopy is an essential adjunct to VATS in the assessment of lung expansion in all patients undergoing VATS. Malignant airway involvement may account for failure to obtain lung expansion at VATS, either as the sole cause or as an additional factor adding to the common cause of malignant lung entrapment (**Fig. 6**).

TUNNELED PLEURAL CATHETERS VERSUS VATS TALC PLEURODESIS

A retrospective study of 109 patients with MPE reported a reduced hospital length of stay for patients palliated with TPC versus VATS talc pleurodesis (mean, 7 days vs 8 days; mode, 1 day vs 4 days, $P = .006$).[23] Criteria for discharge or reasons for prolongation of hospital stay related or unrelated to the procedures were not given. Postprocedure complications, in-hospital mortality, and hospital readmissions were similar between treatment groups. Reintervention for recurrent ipsilateral

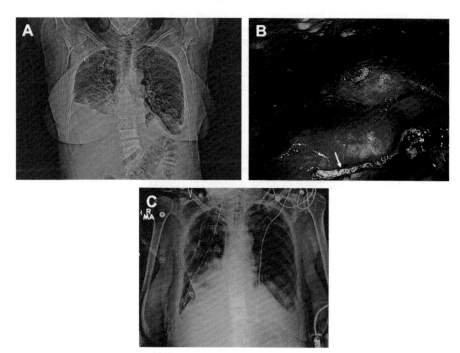

Fig. 9. (*A*) Preprocedure scout computed tomography of a 64-year-old patient with breast cancer, who had failed thoracentesis and bedside chemical pleurodesis but was responding to systemic therapy. It was thought that her survival was greater than 6 months. (*B*) View at VATS decortication including metastasectomy (*arrow*) before talc poudrage. (*C*) Immediate postoperative chest radiograph.

presumably did not include repeated drainage of TPC patients, was less common in the TPC group than in the VATS talc pleurodesis group (2% vs 16%, $P = .01$). Unfortunately, these retrospective data were not analyzed with propensity scoring; without a matching analysis the results are just as easily explained by patient selection as by the different techniques.[24]

DECORTICATION

There is no doubt that pleurectomy and decortication is an effective procedure for controlling the pleural space. However, the morbidity of pleurectomy and decortication at thoracotomy in patients with MPE greatly reduces its palliative benefit. The exception is malignant mesothelioma, in which this surgical option has evolved into the procedure of choice for palliation of MPE complicating mesothelioma. The use of thoracotomy with decortication as primary palliation for all other MPE is of historical interst.[25] Discovery of MPE at thoracotomy during lung cancer resection is ominous. The retrospective literature confirms that resection of lung cancers in this setting should be avoided,[26] particularly with N2 or N3 regional lymph node metastases,[27] but palliation of the MPE or potential MPE is indicated.

Decortication is practiced to some extent at all diagnostic and therapeutic VATS procedures for pleural effusions, be it simple drainage of the fluid and breaking down loculations (**Fig. 7**), adhesiolysis (**Fig. 8**), or partial decortication (**Fig. 9**). Typically, this "quasi" decortication alone is insufficient for palliation, and pleurodesis or an indwelling catheter should be added.

SUMMARY

The surgical management of MPE is a fine balancing act. The patient's wishes, performance status, and prognosis must be weighed alongside the ability to obtain full lung expansion and control fluid production. The benefit of palliation should not be lost during the surgical procedure or recovery from it. With the advent of VATS and TPC, typically "less is more."

REFERENCES

1. Beyea A, Winzelberg G, Stafford RE. To drain or not to drain: an evidence-based approach to palliative procedures for the management of malignant pleural effusions. J Pain Symptom Manage 2012; 44(2):301–6.
2. Musani AI. Treatment options for malignant pleural effusion. Curr Opin Pulm Med 2009;15(4):380–7.
3. factors for survival after surgical palliation of m pleural effusion. J Thorac Oncol 2010;5(10):
4. MacEachern P, Tremblay A. Pleural con pleurodesis versus indwelling pleural cath malignant effusions. Respirology 2011;16(5)
5. Murthy SC, Okereke I, Mason DP, et al. / solution for complicated pleural effusions. Oncol 2006;1(7):697–700.
6. Efthymiou CA, Masudi T, Thorpe JA, et al. N pleural effusion in the presence of trapp Five-year experience of PleurX tunnelled c Interact Cardiovasc Thorac Surg 2009;9(6)
7. Lee P. Point: should thoracoscopic talc pleurc the first choice management for malignant Yes. Chest 2012;142(1):15–7 [discussion: 2(
8. Light RW. Counterpoint: should thoracosc(pleurodesis be the first choice manageı malignant pleural effusion? No. Chest 201 17–9 [discussion: 19–20].
9. Demmy TL, Gu L, Burkhalter JE, et al. management of malignant pleural effusions of CALGB 30102). J Natl Compr Canc Ne 10(8):975–82.
10. Shaw P, Agarwal R. Pleurodesis for m pleural effusions. Cochrane Database S 2004;(1):CD002916.
11. Stefani A, Natali P, Casali C, et al. Talc p versus talc slurry in the treatment of m pleural effusion. A prospective comparativ Eur J Cardiothorac Surg 2006;30(6):827–32
12. Tan C, Sedrakyan A, Browne J, et al. The e on the effectiveness of management for m pleural effusion: a systematic review. Eur J thorac Surg 2006;29(5):829–38.
13. Putnam JB Jr, Light RW, Rodriguez RM A randomized comparison of indwelling catheter and doxycycline pleurodesis management of malignant pleural effusions 1999;86(10):1992–9.
14. Suzuki K, Servais EL, Rizk NP, et al. Pallia pleurodesis in malignant pleural effusion: for tunneled pleural catheters. J Thora(2011;6(4):762–7.
15. Thornton RH, Miller Z, Covey AM, et al. 1 pleural catheters for treatment of recurre nant pleural effusion following failed pleu J Vasc Interv Radiol 2010;21(5):696–700.
16. Janes SM, Rahman NM, Davies RJ, et a eter-tract metastases associated with indwelling pleural catheters. Chest 200; 1232–4.
17. Fysh ET, Wrightson JM, Lee YC, et al. F indwelling pleural catheters. Chest 2012 1090–4.
18. Van Meter ME, McKee KY, Kohlwes RJ. Effic safety of tunneled pleural catheters in ad

malignant pleural effusions: a systematic review. J Gen Intern Med 2011;26(1):70–6.

19. Aelony Y, Yao JF. Prolonged survival after talc poudrage for malignant pleural mesothelioma: case series. Respirology 2005;10(5):649–55.

20. Nasreen N, Mohammed KA, Brown S, et al. Talc mediates angiostasis in malignant pleural effusions via endostatin induction. Eur Respir J 2007;29(4):761–9.

21. Reddy C, Ernst A, Lamb C, et al. Rapid pleurodesis for malignant pleural effusions: a pilot study. Chest 2011;139(6):1419–23.

22. Antunes G, Neville E, Duffy J, et al. BTS guidelines for the management of malignant pleural effusions. Thorax 2003;58(Suppl 2):ii29–38.

23. Hunt BM, Farivar AS, Vallières E, et al. Thoracoscopic talc versus tunneled pleural catheters for palliation of malignant pleural effusions. Ann Thorac Surg 2012;94:1053–9.

24. Blackstone EH. Comparing apples and oranges. J Thorac Cardiovasc Surg 2002;123:8–15.

25. Beattie EJ Jr. The treatment of malignant pleural effusions by parietal pleurectomy. Surg Clin North Am 1963;43:99–108.

26. Sawabata N, Matsumura A, Motohiro A, et al. Malignant minor pleural effusions detected on thoracotomy for patients with non-small cell lung cancer: is tumor resection beneficial for prognosis? Ann Thorac Surg 2002;73:412–5.

27. Okamoto T, Iwata T, Mizobuchi T, et al. Pulmonary resection for lung cancer with malignant pleural disease first detected at thoracotomy. Eur J Cardiothorac Surg 2012;41:25–30.

Pleurectomy Decortication in the Treatment of the "Trapped Lung" in Benign and Malignant Pleural Effusions

Sridhar Rathinam, FRCSEd(CTh)*, David A. Waller, FRCS(CTh)

KEYWORDS

- Pleural effusion • Empyema thoracic • Malignant • Mesothelioma • Decortication
- Video-assisted thoracic surgery

KEY POINTS

- Trapped lung is characterized by the inability of the lung to expand and fill the thoracic cavity because of a restricting "peel," either an inflammatory cortex or visceral pleural tumor.
- The process of peeling of the organized cortex of the visceral pleura from the lung to aid re-expansion of the trapped lung is called decortication.
- In the case of benign pleural effusion, decortication can be safely achieved by VATS. Early intervention with VATS offers the best results and prevents development of thick fibrous cortex.
- Trapped lung caused by mesothelioma, lung cancer, or secondary malignancies is managed by VATS visceral pleurectomy or open extended pleurectomy decortications for relief of dyspnea and possible survival benefit in mesothelioma.
- It is debatable whether VATS visceral pleurectomy is indicated in metastatic disease, where it might be a better option to place pleurex catheters.

INTRODUCTION

Trapped lung is defined by the inability of the lung to expand and fill the thoracic cavity because of a restricting "peel." This restriction may be secondary to a benign inflammatory or fibrotic cortex or to a malignant visceral pleural tumor. Benign causes include progression of a parapneumonic effusion, secondary infection of a postoperative or traumatic hemothorax,[1] or pleural fibrosis. Malignant causes of trapped lung are most commonly malignant pleural mesothelioma (MPM) or metastatic pleural disease.[2]

This condition has a significant impact on the patient's quality of life by causing dyspnea from ventilatory restriction and ventilation: perfusion mismatch compounded by the constitutional effects of an inflammatory process or malignant disease.

This article discusses the role of surgery in relieving the trapped lung including decortication in benign disease and pleurectomy in malignant disease. The surgical approaches of video-assisted thoracoscopy (VATS) and thoracotomy are contrasted and the future potential for surgical trials in this condition is outlined.

SURGICAL ANATOMY OF THE PLEURA

The pleural cavity of the thorax is lined by the parietal and visceral pleura. The visceral pleura is in close apposition to the lung surfaces and lines the major and minor fissures of the lungs. The parietal pleura lines the chest wall, the diaphragm, and the mediastinum, and forms the pleural dome at the thoracic inlet. The diaphragmatic pleura and mediastinal pleura adhere tightly to the diaphragm

Department of Thoracic Surgery, Glenfield Hospital, University Hospitals of Leicester, Groby Road, Leicester, LE3 9QP, UK
* Corresponding author.
E-mail address: srathinam@rcsed.ac.uk

Thorac Surg Clin 23 (2013) 51–61
http://dx.doi.org/10.1016/j.thorsurg.2012.10.007

and the pericardium, but have a cleavage plane in the remainder of the mediastinal pleura, the inlets, and the costal pleura, where it can be readily dissected from the underlying tissues.[3]

PATHOPHYSIOLOGY

The pleural space is a potential space that contains pleural fluid, which lubricates the pleura and facilitates lung expansion and protects the lung. Pleural effusion of any cause leads to accumulation of fluid in this space, which compromises respiratory function. As the condition persists and progresses and the pleura forms a thick cortex, it further compromises respiratory dynamics by impeding chest wall movements and lung expansion. The symptoms of dyspnea may also be compounded by ventilation-perfusion mismatch within the entrapped lobe or lobes.

IMAGING OF THE TRAPPED LUNG
Chest Radiography

After complete drainage of a pleural effusion a chest radiograph may give the first indication of entrapment of the underlying lung and may give an impression of a thickened visceral cortex (**Fig. 1**).

Ultrasonography

Thoracic ultrasonography can identify empyemas and hemorrhagic effusions by echogenicity and septation. Transudates are always anechoic, but exudates may also be anechoic. Effusions are usually exudates when they are septated or show a complex or homogeneously echogenic pattern.[4] Unfortunately, ultrasound is not reliable in identifying whether the underlying lung is entrapped.

Computed Tomography

Computed tomography (CT) is useful in illustrating the status of the underlying lung. Contrast-enhanced CT can identify parietal pleural thickening in empyema and parapneumonic effusions (**Fig. 2**). However, it is not possible to estimate the thickness of the visceral cortex because this may be falsely thickened by the overlying exudate and debris.

Because imaging cannot reliably identify those patients who require surgical intervention for a trapped lung after failed management by chest tube drainage and intrapleural fibrinolytics[5] initial assessment by VATS is recommended in all cases. It is important to drain a malignant effusion to dryness to determine whether or not the lung will expand. It is very important to avoid repeated interventions (ie, aspiration) to reduce the risk of malignant empyema.

TRAPPED LUNG IN BENIGN PLEURAL DISEASE

Empyema thoracis is a dynamic process in which purulent effusion or pus accumulates in the pleural space from various causes, localized or involving the entire pleural cavity. The incidence of empyema continues to increase and still causes significant morbidity and mortality.[6]

Empyema can be classified as intrinsic or extrinsic depending on the causative process. Extrinsic thoracic empyema results from such causes as surgery, instrumentation, and penetrating and blunt chest trauma. Intrinsic empyema occurs when there is no previous surgical intervention to the chest, in most cases because of postpneumonic or parapneumonic effusions and tuberculous effusions. The most common form of empyema thoracis

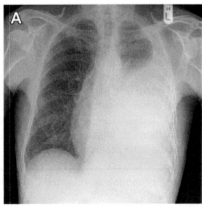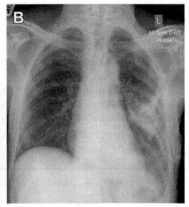

Fig. 1. (*A*) Chest radiograph demonstrating a large left-sided pleural effusion in a 78 year old with progressive shortness of breath. (*B*) Chest radiograph demonstrating a trapped unexpanded lung after drainage of the left-sided pleural effusion.

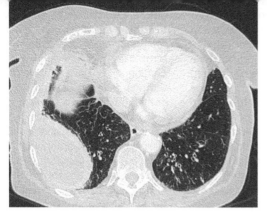

Fig. 2. CT scan demonstrating a large pleural effusion with trapped lung.

is postpneumonic or parapneumonic effusions (40%–60%), followed by thoracic surgical procedures (30%), and then post traumatic empyemas.[7–9]

Causative Organisms

Before the antibiotic era *Streptococcus pneumoniae* was the most frequent causative organism, but now *Staphylococcus aureus* is the most common organism causing empyema.[10] Community-acquired infections are usually gram-positive organisms; most are streptococcal, of which *Streptococcus milleri* is the most common. In about 15% of cases anaerobic cultures are positive, associated with poor dentition and aspiration. Hospital-acquired infections are mostly gram-negative; 25% of all nosocomial infections in the United Kingdom are methicillin-resistant *Staphylococcus aureus* (MRSA). *Enterococcus*, *Enterobacteriaceae* (30%), and *Staphylococcus* spp are isolated in 18% of cases.

Pathology

The progression of postpneumonic effusion to organized empyema manifests in a phased manner over a 3- to 6-week period. This was stratified by the American Thoracic Society into three stages as the exudative stage 1, the fibrinopurulent and loculated stage 2, and the more chronic organizational phase of stage 3.[11]

The progression of an untreated empyema leads to trapping of the lung and restriction of chest wall movements. If untreated this eventually leads to a thick fibrinitic layer encasing the lung and chest wall, which eventually fibroses leading to a solid "fibrothorax."[12]

Surgery is indicated when chest drainage and antibiotic treatment have failed to achieve resolution. Trapped lung is a common result of inadequately treated parapneumonic effusion, but it is also associated with cardiac surgery, chest trauma, and other inflammatory processes involving the pleura.[13] It is characterized by inability of the lung to expand and fill the thoracic cavity because of a restricting fibrous visceral pleural peel.

The basic principles of management include drainage of the infected empyema and obliteration of the space to promote symphysis of the lung and chest wall.[14] Decortication is a time honored technique first described by Fowler in 1893[15] and later by DeLorme,[14] which was traditionally used for the treatment of tuberculous and posttraumatic trapped lung.[9,16] It relies on lung elasticity to fill the cavity, having freed the encased parenchyma from the compressing cortex.

In chronic empyemas, particularly in stage 3 disease, with a history of more than 6 weeks, if the patient is fit for surgery they benefit from open decortication.[17,18] Timing is the cornerstone of surgical judgment allowing the "rind to mature," but preventing the onset of a fixed fibrothorax.

SURGICAL APPROACH TO DECORTICATION

Thoracotomy was the mainstay treatment option until the advent of thoracoscopic debridement and decortication toward the end of the twentieth century.[19–22]

Technique

Preoperative bronchoscopy should be performed to exclude endobronchial obstruction caused by sputum, inhaled foreign body, or tumor.

Thoracotomy and Decortication (Empyemectomy)

It is performed under general anesthesia using single lung ventilation. Access is through a lateral thoracotomy or posterolateral thoracotomy. Often it is necessary to create an extrapleural plane to perform the thoracotomy because of the fibrinous nature of the parietal pleura. The purpose of removing the thickened peel over the surface of the lung is so that it can re-expand and the pleural surfaces can be reopposed, eliminating the potential space that harbors bacteria. The principle of surgery is complete removal of the pleural abscess cavity (empyemectomy) and restoration of chest wall mechanics and re-expansion of lung. After parietal decortication is performed the junction of the visceral cortex with the unaffected

visceral pleura is entered by sharp or blunt dissection until normal lung is felt proceeding to the identification of tissue plane between the abscess wall
and visceral pleura. It is helpful to have positive
pressure applied to the operated lung because
this provides counter pressure while dissecting
the cortex away from the lung. If the lung is very
friable or in the absence of an adequate plane to
decorticate the visceral pleura it is possible to
perform incisions into the visceral pleura, either
in a parallel fashion or in a checkerboard fashion,
to allow the lung to re-expand as described by
Ransohoff in 1900. However, this technique is
associated with greater postoperative air leak.

It is important to achieve adequate pneumosta-
sis and hemostasis at the end of the operation.
Parenchymal injuries are surgically repaired with
sutures or by excising them with staplers. Airleaks
can also be controlled by the use of glues, sealants, and aerosols adhesives. Likewise, hemostasis can be aided by the use of hemostasis
sealants. It is imperative to ensure meticulous
hemostasis because the chronicity of the condition may have resulted in extensive vascular adhesions to the cortex. Thorough decortication is
recommended to ensure full re-expansion of the
affected lung. This facilitates tamponade of postoperative air leak and bleeding.

VATS Decortication

VATS is performed under general anesthesia with
single lung ventilation and the patient in lateral decubitus position. A 2-cm incision just inferior and
anterior to the inferior angle of the scapula is
made through which the thoracoscope is inserted
after freeing the adhesions by digital exploration.
Alternatively, the first port site is placed in the
fourth intercostal space in the anterior axillary
line, at a site distant to the area of pleural collection
to facilitate entry into the thoracic cavity. The
remaining two incisions are placed in the line of
the same intercostal space, usually the sixth or
seventh, and the dissecting instruments are inserted under video guidance. A simple effusion
can be drained by suction at this stage. The other
two ports are placed under direct vision to avoid
injury to vessels or lung. The contents are evacuated by suction and blunt dissection. Initial pleural
debridement is performed using directed suction
with a modified 36F catheter gauge intercostal
tube combined with saline lavage. The parietal
pleura is dissected by sharp and blunt dissection
from the chest wall and diaphragm taking particular care at the apices.

An assessment is then made of the ability to
re-expand the underlying lung by ventilation to

a positive pressure of 40 cm H2O. If the lu
not re-expand under direct vision, beca
the thick inflammatory peel that preven
re-expansion, then a visceral decortication
formed. To facilitate removal of the viscera
continuous positive airways pressure is ap
the operative lung during dissection. The
continuous positive airways pressure is
and dictated by the restricted space wit
hemithorax. After mechanical breakdown o
sions and septae aided with regular saline
outs an initial incision is made in the v
cortex using endoscopic shears and proc
in a radial direction across the lateral as
the trapped lobe. The correct surgical p
accessed by sharply incising the visceral
and this layer is carefully peeled off fr
underlying lung using blunt dissectio
the aid of a mounted pledget or the blunt
the yankeur sucker (**Fig. 3**). By graspi
edge of the cortex the plane between it a
visceral pleura, the elevated cortical s
then removed by a combination of tracti
rolling. Care is taken to clear the cortex fr
fissures to ensure complete re-expansi
identify isolated pockets of sepsis in the
The pleural cavity is then washed with
with or without aqueous betadine. If the
any pockets of air leaks aerosolized fibr
can be sprayed onto the lung surface. Inte
drains are placed to drain the chest. VA
empyema may be converted to open dec
tion in 4% to 40% of cases depending
stage of empyema.[23]

Alternative Management

If it is not possible to perform decorticati
attempts to obliterate the pleural space
made by interposing muscle flaps or co
the chest wall (thoracoplasty). If all these me
fail then the space can be drained to the cut
surface by thoracostomy window.[24,25]

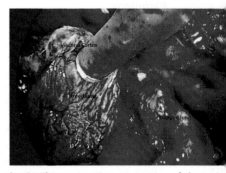

Fig. 3. Thoracoscopic appearance of decortic
visceral pleural cortex in empyema with blun
tion with pledget mounted widebore drain.

RESULTS OF DECORTICATION FOR BENIGN TRAPPED LUNG

Open Decortication

Decortication is a highly effective treatment for chronic parapneumonic empyema and may be performed with low morbidity and mortality. The outcomes of surgical decortication are dependent on the duration of preoperative treatments, comorbidities, and preoperative duration of symptoms-predicted morbidity.[26,27]

Surgical decortication is associated with varied morbidity and mortality given the coexisting sepsis and comorbidities. Decortication is more frequently necessary for anaerobic, tuberculous, staphylococcal, and pneumococcal infections.[28] Surgical decortication achieves a better success rate compared with conservative management options.[29] In overall care and outcomes, surgical decortication also was cost effective by the virtue of a reduced procedure failure rate or failed therapeutic option.[18] 80% of post traumatic empyema requires formal decortication and have very good outcomes.[8]

Chronic empyema traps the lung, reduces the lung capacity, and reduces lung perfusion to the involved side. Releasing the trapped lung improves pulmonary perfusion and improves forced vital capacity (FVC) from 61% up to 77% and forced expiratory volume in 1 second (FEV1) from 61% to 78%.[30,31] Its value has been demonstrated in decortication of trapped lung in tuberculous empyema.[32] Similar improvement is seen after decortication to release trapped lung in patients after cardiac surgery with improvement in their dyspnea score and lung capacity. The mean preoperative FEV1 and FVC, which were $63.8\% \pm 7.4\%$ and $50.5\% \pm 6.6\%$ of the predicted value, respectively, improved by a rate of $14.97\% \pm 6.3\%$ and $17.62\% \pm 6.38\%$, respectively.[33]

VATS Decortication

VATS decortication is a feasible treatment of chronic pleural empyema when pleural debridement alone is insufficient. Using conventional instruments it is a safe, effective, and durable method of achieving re-expansion of the trapped underlying lung by removing the visceral cortex in the same way as in open surgery.[19,23,34] VATS surgical decortication has higher treatment success, lower chest tube duration, and decreased total hospital days compared with tube thoracostomy alone.

Various authors have reported success with VATS decortication for empyema of mixed stage (stages 2/3) with the conversion rate ranging from 7.1% to 17% with operative mortality of 0% to 6.6%. The postoperative stay was variable with a range of 7.4 ± 7.2 to 5 ± 0.7 days.[19,35,36]

VATS decortication used in the treatment of complicated parapneumonic effusion (stage 2) (N = 145) and loculated empyema (stage 3) (N = 89) showed there was significant reductions in postoperative length of stay (stage 2, 9.1 vs stage 3, 18.5 days; $P<0.05$), perioperative morbidity (effusion, 6.2% vs empyema, 11.2%; $P<0.05$) and perioperative mortality (effusion, 2.1% vs empyema, 5.6%; $P<0.05$).[37]

The success of VATS decortication depends on the stage of the empyema. Outcomes have steadily improved with growing experience of the technique.[38,39] There is evidence that earlier intervention with VATS decortication has a better outcome. VATS decortication in stage 2 resulted in lesser conversion rate, decreased morbidity and mortality, and lesser hospital length of stay.

Which Approach is Preferable?

VATS decortication when compared with open decortication has been reported to have shorter operative time (2.5 vs 3.8 h; $P<0.001$); lesser postoperative pain ($P = 0.04$); greater satisfaction with the wounds ($P<0.0001$); and greater satisfaction with the operation overall ($P = 0.006$).[40] VATS decortication had reduced hospital stays (15 vs 21 days; $P = 0.03$) and significantly reduced postoperative complications and 30-day mortality in a study of 420 patients ($P = 0.02$).[41] It also reduced operative time, pain, postoperative air leak, hospital stay, and time to return to work when compared with open decortication for chronic empyema.[23,42]

VAT decortication has many postoperative benefits over open surgery in the long term.[43] Patients have a shorter period of general anesthesia because of the time saved in avoiding opening and closure of the thoracotomy. The length of stay is reduced in comparison with open surgery because of reduced requirement for invasive pain control (thoracic epidural) and earlier mobilization.[23] A proportion of patients undergoing VATS approach for empyema are likely to be converted to thoracotomy and decortication (3.8% to 40%) depending on the delay in decision even as early as stage 2.[37–39] The advantage of thoracotomy is the reduction in reoperation rate after initial treatment failure, which is half of that after VATS procedure. However, the current practice is to attempt VATS first and convert it to a thoracotomy if success is not achieved during the same anesthesia.

The latest progress in this area is "awake" video-assisted pleural decortication. In this technique the patient remains spontaneously ventilated under sedation during VATS. Initial reports are promising with satisfactory lung re-expansion in 95% of patients.[44]

TRAPPED LUNG IN MALIGNANT PLEURAL DISEASE

In contrast to benign pleural disease, in these cases the entrapment is secondary to malignant infiltration and thickening of the visceral pleura itself. There may also be a secondary infective cortex but the principles of surgical therapy involve visceral pleurectomy rather than just decortication. The surgical plane is therefore one layer lower exposing the underlying lung parenchyma. Visceral pleurectomy is offered with intentional therapeutic and palliative benefit because it is viewed as potential cytoreduction.

Malignant Empyema

Inappropriate repeated pleural intervention in a malignant pleural effusion may result in an infected space and the development of an empyema. This is the worst of both worlds for the patient. They have the detrimental systemic effects of advanced malignancy and chronic infection. Their generally poor condition usually precludes extended pleurectomy and decortication (EPD) and thoracostomy drainage may be all that is feasible.

Underlying Malignancy

The entrapped lung may be caused by primary malignancy of the visceral pleura (ie, malignant pleural mesothelioma), which is commonly broken down into three histologic subtypes: (1) epithelioid, (2) sarcomatoid, and (3) biphasic. The visceral pleura may also be infiltrated by metastatic tumor from a distant primary. The most common sites are lung, breast, colon, and ovary.[45]

Surgical Strategies

Prior knowledge of the histologic diagnosis of the underlying malignancy influences the choice of operative technique. The role of visceral pleurectomy in metastatic disease is likely to be of less benefit than in malignant mesothelioma. In surgery of mesothelioma there are three contrasting options: EPD or partial pleurectomy by either VATS or video-assisted thoracotomy.

Visceral Pleurectomy in Malignant Mesothelioma

Extended pleurectomy and decortication

An entrapped lung does not preclude EPD.[46] This operation entails macroscopic complete resection with total visceral and parietal pleurectomy with en bloc excision of the pericardium and diaphragm if necessary. It is suitable for all cell types but the results in sarcomatoid mesothelioma are disappointing and are probably no better than palliative procedures.[47] In general if a patient is considered fit enough to undergo a lobectomy for lung cancer then they are fit enough for an EPD. Survival after EPD is very similar to that after the more extensive extrapleural pneumonectomy but associated mortality and morbidity are reduced.[48] EPD can also be performed in bulky stage III mesothelioma with achievement of macroscopic complete resection.[49]

Open partial pleurectomy

In the case of malignant pleural effusions it is important to consider the expected survival and prognosis before venturing into surgery for trapped lung. In patients with an expected survival of less than 12 months it is probably not appropriate to perform a thoracotomy, which may have a 3-month recovery. Therefore, if partial pleurectomy is considered for symptom relief of the malignant trapped lung it is best to use a video-assisted approach. If open surgery is considered then it should be with the intention of more significant life prolongation and therefore be an EPD with macroscopic complete resection.[50]

VATS pleurectomy and decortication

VATS parietal pleurectomy has been shown to offer palliation and effects good symptom control.[51,52] The technique has been extended to the visceral surface with good effect.[53] It involves a similar technique to VATS decortication of empyema but the lung parenchyma must be exposed (**Figs. 4** and **5**). The importance of obtaining good lung re-expansion by persisting with the visceral pleurectomy cannot be overemphasized. Only by achieving lung apposition with the pleura can a prolonged air leak be prevented.

VATS pleurectomy and decortication was initially reserved for older and less fit patients who were unfit for a radical procedure (extra pleural pneumonectomy (EPP) or EPD). With increasing experience EPD is being offered to more elderly patients (older than 75 years) but the benefits of EPD over VATS pleurectomy and decortication seem less evident in nonepithelioid malignant pleural mesothelioma (MPM) and in those with nodal metastatic disease.[53,54] Other benefits of VATS total pleurectomy include a reduction in the number of misdiagnosed MPM cases.[55] Visceral pleural decortication improves diagnosis and symptoms in patients with MPM[56] and may have superior long-term survival to biopsy and pleurodesis alone.[57] It can alleviate symptoms and seems to prolong survival, but further research is needed to assess its role in the management of malignant pleural mesothelioma (**Table 1**).[58]

Table 1
Outcomes after decortication for malignant effusion

Series	Total Number	Surgical Intent	VATS Pleurectomy	End Point	Outcome	Conclusion
Waller et al,[52] 1995 UK Cohort Study	19 patients 13 malignant mesothelioma, 6 metastatic adenocarcinoma	Palliation	All	Postoperative stay	Median 5 d (2–20 d)	VATS parietal pleurectomy safe and effective palliative measure if visceral pleura is not heavily diseased
				Recurrence of effusion Survival	2 patients 6 died of disease process (2 mesothelioma) At median of 4 mo (2–8 mo)	
Grossebner et al,[56] 1999 UK cohort study	25 patients 23 mesothelioma Pleural symphisis achieved in 15	Diagnosis Cyto reduction and palliation	All	Air leak	Median 5 d (2–12 d)	VATS provides for adequate histologic diagnosis and therapeutic intervention
				Recurrence of effusion Survival	1 patient Pleurectomy and symphisis: 11 patients at 1–2 y No pleural symphisis 1 alive at 9 mo (rest died within 6 mo)	
Martin-Ucar et al,[51] 2001 UK cohort study	51 patients with advanced MPM	Palliative drainage, lung re-expansion, pleurodesis, and debulking Releasing entrapped lung	VATS parietal pleurectomy: N = 17 VATS parietal and visceral pleurectomy N = 3 Thoracotomy and parietal and visceral pleurectomy N = 31	Prolonged Air leak Length of stay Survival	5 (9.8%) 7 d (2–17 d) 89% at 6 wk, 71% at 3 mo, 56% at 6 mo and 31% at 12 mo	Type of procedure did not significantly influence survival (P = 0.07) There were benefits from debulking surgery including by VATS

(continued on next page)

Table 1
(continued)

Series	Total Number	Surgical Intent	VATS Pleurectomy	End Point	Outcome	Conclusion
Halstead et al,[57] 2005 UK cohort study	79 patients with advanced MPM		28 underwent VATS biopsy 51 had VATS pleurectomy decortication	Actuarial survival	Biopsy group vs 127 d Pleurectomy decortication group: 416 d $P<0.001$	VATS pleurectomy decortication is feasible in most patients and improves survival in advanced MPM
				Prolonged air leak	Biopsy group: 57% 84% for pleurectomy decortication group: 84% $P = 0.01$	
				Length of stay	Biopsy group 4 d Pleurectomy decortication group: 8 d $P = 0.03$	
Nakas et al,[53] 2008 UK cohort study	208 patients had therapeutic surgery for MPM over a 9-year period. Of which 63 patients older than 65 y were analyzed	Curative intent Palliation to expand trapped lung in unfit patients	EPP = 13 Pleurectomy decortications: 8 VATS decortications: 42	Postoperative stay	EPP: 36.6 d (9–184) Thoracotomy pleurectomy and decortication: 14 d (9–24) VATS decortication 14.3 d (10–28) $P<0.05$	58% improvement in pain and 83% improvement in dyspnea in VATS pleurectomy and decortication group and suggests that VATS decortication is an effective palliation method in patients >70 y old
				30-day mortality	EPP: 3 (23%) Thoracotomy pleurectomy and decortication: 1 (12.5%) VATS decortication 3 (7.5%) $P<0.05$	
				Overall mean survival	EPP: 11.5 mo Thoracotomy PD: 12.5 mo VATS decortication: 14 mo	

Abbreviations: EPP, Extra Pleural Pneumonectomy; MPM, Malignant Pleural Mesothelioma; VATS, Video assisted thoracoscopic surgery.

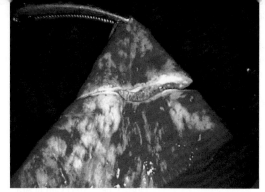

Fig. 4. Incision of visceral pleura in VATS pleural decortication in malignant mesothelioma.

Physiologic Benefits of Visceral Pleurectomy

Debulking of malignant mesothelioma with pleurectomy decortication substantially increased the ipsilateral lung volume relative to the presurgical ipsilateral volume and the contralateral lung volume. This improvement persisted months after surgery.[59] Lung-sparing radical pleurectomy leads to significant improvement of pulmonary function and perfusion particularly in patients where the diaphragm was preserved.[60]

FUTURE WORK

The MesoVATS study in the United Kingdom was designed to address the value of VATS pleurectomy with conventional talc pleurodesis for treatment of pleural effusion in patients with MPM with endpoints of 1-year survival, control of effusion, and quality of life. The study has closed recruiting with results awaited. Unfortunately, patients with trapped lung were excluded from

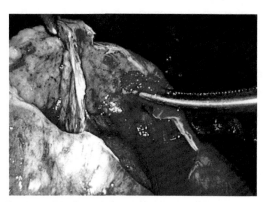

Fig. 5. VATS visceral decortication involves entering a plane between the inelastic fibrous rind and true visceral pleura.

this study but the implications of the results for surgical debulking are awaited.

The role of EPD is to be assessed in the proposed MARS2 (Mesothelioma and Radical Surgery) study in which patients will be randomized to chemotherapy followed by EPD or no surgery. The analysis will focus on quality of life and survival differences.

SUMMARY

Trapped lung is characterized by the inability of the lung to expand and fill the thoracic cavity because of a restricting "peel," either an inflammatory cortex or visceral pleural tumor. Postpneumonic empyema causes trapped lung when the there is an organized inflammatory pleural cortex encasing the lung. Empyemas can be managed by "empyemectomy," which is removal of the empyema cavity intact by dissecting in the plane between the visceral pleura and inflammatory cortex. Decortication involves freeing the cortex from the lung and chest wall to achieve re-expansion of the lung and restore chest wall mechanics. Decortication can be safely achieved by VATS surgery. Early intervention for benign pleural effusions and empyemas with thoracoscopic approach offers the best results and prevents development of thick fibrous cortex and therefore the need for decortication.

Malignant visceral pleural tumor can cause trapped lung in malignant pleural mesothelioma or metastatic malignancy most commonly caused by lung cancer. The two strategic options are VATS visceral pleurectomy for relief of dyspnea and possible survival benefit or open EPD. There is no place for open partial pleurectomy because the patient's terminal life is spent recovering from the thoracotomy. If one commits to a thoracotomy all visible tumor should be removed (macroscopic complete resection). It is debatable whether VATS visceral pleurectomy is indicated in metastatic disease (where prognosis is poor). It might be a better option to place PleurX catheters in these situations. EPD has many benefits over extrapulmonary pneumonectomy, such as better quality of life, better lung perfusion, and spirometry with available evidence suggesting comparative or better survival.

REFERENCES

1. Doelken P, Sahn SA. Trapped lung. Semin Respir Crit Care Med 2001;22(6):631–6.
2. Lombardi G, Zustovich F, Nicoletto MO, et al. Diagnosis and treatment of malignant pleural effusion: a systematic literature review and new approaches. Am J Clin Oncol 2010;33(4):420–3.

3. Bertin F, Deslauriers J. Anatomy of the pleura: reflection lines and recesses. Thorac Surg Clin 2011; 21(2):165–71, vii.

4. Yang PC, Luh KT, Chang DB, et al. Value of sonography in determining the nature of pleural effusion: analysis of 320 cases. AJR Am J Roentgenol 1992;159(1):29–33.

5. Kearney SE, Davies CW, Davies RJ, et al. Computed tomography and ultrasound in parapneumonic effusions and empyema. Clin Radiol 2000;55(7):542–7.

6. Lee SF, Lawrence D, Booth H, et al. Thoracic empyema: current opinions in medical and surgical management. Curr Opin Pulm Med 2010;16(3): 194–200.

7. de Hoyos A, Sundaresan S. Thoracic empyema. Surg Clin North Am 2002;82(3):643–71, viii.

8. Mandal AK, Thadepalli H, Mandal AK, et al. Posttraumatic empyema thoracis: a 24-year experience at a major trauma center. J Trauma 1997;43(5):764–71.

9. Molnar TF. Current surgical treatment of thoracic empyema in adults. Eur J Cardiothorac Surg 2007; 32(3):422–30.

10. Ozol D, Oktem S, Erdinc E. Complicated parapneumonic effusion and empyema thoracis: microbiologic and therapeutic aspects. Respir Med 2006; 100(2):286–91.

11. Andrews NC. Management of nontuberculous empyema: a statement of the subcommittee on surgery. Am Rev Respir Dis 1962;85935.

12. Jantz MA, Antony VB. Pleural fibrosis. Clin Chest Med 2006;27(2):181–91.

13. Doelken P. Clinical implications of unexpandable lung due to pleural disease. Am J Med Sci 2008; 335(1):21–5.

14. DeLorme E. Nouveau traitment des empyémes chroniques. Gaz d Hop 1894;67:94–6.

15. Fowler GR. A case of thoracoplasty for the removal of a large cicatricial fibrous growth from the interior of the chest, the result of an old empyema. New York Med Rec 1893;44:638–839.

16. Samson PC, Burford TH. Total pulmonary decortications. Its evaluation and present concepts of indication and operative technique. J Thorac Surg 1947; 16(2):127–53.

17. Anstadt MP, Guill CK, Ferguson ER, et al. Surgical versus nonsurgical treatment of empyema thoracis: an outcomes analysis. Am J Med Sci 2003;326(1):9–14.

18. Thourani VH, Brady KM, Mansour KA, et al. Evaluation of treatment modalities for thoracic empyema: a cost-effectiveness analysis. Ann Thorac Surg 1998;66(4):1121–7.

19. Landreneau RJ, Keenan RJ, Hazelrigg SR, et al. Thoracoscopy for empyema and hemothorax. Chest 1996;109(1):18–24.

20. Silen ML, Naunheim KS. Thoracoscopic approach to the management of empyema thoracis. Indications and results. Chest Surg Clin N Am 1996;6(3):491–9.

21. Striffeler H, Ris HB, Wursten HU, et al. Video-assisted thoracoscopic treatment of pleural empyema. A new therapeutic approach. Eur J Cardiothorac Surg 1994;8(11):585–8.

22. Waller DA. Thoracoscopy in management of pneumonic pleural infections. Curr Opin Pulm Med 2002;8(4):323–6.

23. Waller DA, Rengarajan A. Thoracoscopic decortication: a role for video-assisted surgery in postpneumonic pleural empyema. Ann Thorac Surg 2001;71(6):1813–6.

24. Deslauriers J, Jacques LF, Gregoire J. Role of Eloesser flap and thoracoplasty in the third millennium. Chest Surg Clin N Am 2002;12(3):605.

25. Eloesser L. An operation for tuberculous empyema. 1935. Chest 2009;136(Suppl 5):e30.

26. Andrade-Alegre R, Garisto JD, Zebede S. Open thoracotomy and decortication for chronic empyema. Clinics (Sao Paulo) 2008;63(6):789–93.

27. Melloni G, Carretta A, Ciriaco P, et al. Decortication for chronic parapneumonic empyema: results of a prospective study. World J Surg 2004;28(5)

28. Mandal AK, Thadepalli H, Mandal AK, et al. Outcome of primary empyema thoracis: therapeutic and microbiologic aspects. Ann Thorac Surg 1998; 66(5):1782–6.

29. LeMense GP, Strange C, Sahn SA. Empyema thoracis. Therapeutic management and outcome. Chest 1995;107(6):1532–7.

30. Gokce M, Okur E, Baysungur V, et al. Lung decortication for chronic empaema: effects on pulmonary function and thoracic asymmetry in the late period. Eur J Cardiothorac Surg 2009;36(4):754–8.

31. Rzyman W, Skokowski J, Romanowicz G, et al. Lung function in patients operated for chronic empyema. Thorac Cardiovasc Surg 2005;53(4)

32. Yang HC, Han J, Lee S, et al. Evaluation of decortication in patients with chronic tuberculous empyema by three-dimensional computed tomography densitometry. Thorac Cardiovasc Surg [Epub ahead of print].

33. Celik S, Celik M, Aydemir B, et al. Long-term results of lung decortication in patients with trapped lung secondary to coronary artery bypass grafting. Thorac Cardiovasc Surg 2012;18(2):109–14.

34. Chambers A, Routledge T, Dunning J, et al. Is video-assisted thoracoscopic surgical decortication superior to open surgery in the management of adults with primary empyema? Interact Cardiovasc Thorac Surg 2010;11(2):171–7.

35. Kim BY, Oh BS, Jang WC, et al. Video-assisted thoracoscopic decortication for management of postpneumonic pleural empyema. Am J Surg 2004; 188(3):321–4.

36. Solaini L, Prusciano F, di FF, et al. Video-assisted thoracoscopic treatment in pleural empyema. Minerva Chir 2000;55(12):829–33 [in Italian].

37. Luh SP, Chou MC, Wang LS, et al. Video-assisted thoracoscopic surgery in the treatment of complicated parapneumonic effusions or empyemas: outcome of 234 patients. Chest 2005;127(4):1427–32.

38. Lardinois D, Gock M, Pezzetta E, et al. Delayed referral and gram-negative organisms increase the conversion thoracotomy rate in patients undergoing video-assisted thoracoscopic surgery for empyema. Ann Thorac Surg 2005;79(6): 1851–6.

39. Waller DA, Rengarajan A, Nicholson FH, et al. Delayed referral reduces the success of video-assisted thoracoscopic debridement for post-pneumonic empyema. Respir Med 2001;95(10):836–40.

40. Chan DT, Sihoe AD, Chan S, et al. Surgical treatment for empyema thoracis: is video-assisted thoracic surgery "better" than thoracotomy? Ann Thorac Surg 2007;84(1):225–31.

41. Tong BC, Hanna J, Toloza EM, et al. Outcomes of video-assisted thoracoscopic decortication. Ann Thorac Surg 2010;89(1):220–5.

42. Cardillo G, Carleo F, Carbone L, et al. Chronic post-pneumonic pleural empyema: comparative merits of thoracoscopic versus open decortication. Eur J Cardiothorac Surg 2009;36(5):914–8.

43. Casali C, Storelli ES, Di PE, et al. Long-term functional results after surgical treatment of parapneumonic thoracic empyema. Interact Cardiovasc Thorac Surg 2009;9(1):74–8.

44. Tacconi F, Pompeo E, Fabbi E, et al. Awake video-assisted pleural decortication for empyema thoracis. Eur J Cardiothorac Surg 2010;37(3):594–601.

45. Fry WA, Khandekar JD. Parietal pleurectomy for malignant pleural effusion. Ann Surg Oncol 1995; 2(2):160–4.

46. Rice D, Rusch V, Pass H, et al. Recommendations for uniform definitions of surgical techniques for malignant pleural mesothelioma: a consensus report of the International Association for the Study of Lung Cancer International Staging Committee and the International Mesothelioma Interest Group. J Thorac Oncol 2011;6(8):1304–12.

47. Balduyck B, Trousse D, Nakas A, et al. Therapeutic surgery for nonepithelioid malignant pleural mesothelioma: is it really worthwhile? Ann Thorac Surg 2010;89(3):907–11.

48. Flores RM, Pass HI, Seshan VE, et al. Extrapleural pneumonectomy versus pleurectomy/decortication in the surgical management of malignant pleural mesothelioma: results in 663 patients. J Thorac Cardiovasc Surg 2008;135(3):620–6, 626.

49. Nakas A, von ME, Lau K, et al. Long-term survival after lung-sparing total pleurectomy for locally advanced (International Mesothelioma Interest Group Stage T3-T4) non-sarcomatoid malignant pleural mesothelioma. Eur J Cardiothorac Surg 2012;41(5): 1031–6.

50. Nakas A, Trousse DS, Martin-Ucar AE, et al. Open lung-sparing surgery for malignant pleural mesothelioma: the benefits of a radical approach within multimodality therapy. Eur J Cardiothorac Surg 2008; 34(4):886–91.

51. Martin-Ucar AE, Edwards JG, Rengajaran A, et al. Palliative surgical debulking in malignant mesothelioma. Predictors of survival and symptom control. Eur J Cardiothorac Surg 2001;20(6): 1117–21.

52. Waller DA, Morritt GN, Forty J. Video-assisted thoracoscopic pleurectomy in the management of malignant pleural effusion. Chest 1995;107(5): 1454–6.

53. Nakas A, Martin Ucar AE, Edwards JG, et al. The role of video assisted thoracoscopic pleurectomy/decortication in the therapeutic management of malignant pleural mesothelioma. Eur J Cardiothorac Surg 2008;33(1):83–8.

54. Nakas, Waller DA. Is there any benefit in lung sparing macroscopic complete resection over video assisted debulking in malignant pleural mesothelioma? Proceedings of International Mesothelioma Interest Group Meeting. Boston:2012. p. 83.

55. Hasegawa S, Kondo N, Matsumoto S, et al. Practical approaches to diagnose and treat for T0 malignant pleural mesothelioma: a proposal for diagnostic total parietal pleurectomy. Int J Clin Oncol 2012;17(1):33–9.

56. Grossebner MW, Arifi AA, Goddard M, et al. Mesothelioma–VATS biopsy and lung mobilization improves diagnosis and palliation. Eur J Cardiothorac Surg 1999;16(6):619–23.

57. Halstead JC, Lim E, Venkateswaran RM, et al. Improved survival with VATS pleurectomy-decortication in advanced malignant mesothelioma. Eur J Surg Oncol 2005;31(3):314–20.

58. Srivastava V, Dunning J, Au J. Does video-assisted thoracoscopic decortication in advanced malignant mesothelioma improve prognosis? Interact Cardiovasc Thorac Surg 2009;8(4):454–6.

59. Sensakovic WF, Armato SG III, Starkey A, et al. Quantitative measurement of lung reexpansion in malignant pleural mesothelioma patients undergoing pleurectomy/decortication. Acad Radiol 2011;18(3):294–8.

60. Bolukbas S, Eberlein M, Schirren J. Prospective study on functional results after lung-sparing radical pleurectomy in the management of malignant pleural mesothelioma. J Thorac Oncol 2012;7(5): 900–5.

Permanent Indwelling Catheters in the Management of Pleural Effusions

Jacob Gillen, MD[a], Christine Lau, MD, MBA[b],*

KEYWORDS

- Pleural effusion • Indwelling catheter • PleurX • Lung cancer

KEY POINTS

- Indwelling pleural catheters (IPCs) are being used increasingly as first-line therapy for the treatment of chronic pleural effusions.
- The ideal patient for an IPC has a pleural effusion that recurs in less than 1 month, has a relatively short life expectancy (months), and is a poor surgical candidate.
- Advantages of IPCs over talc pleurodesis include a less invasive outpatient procedure, no requirement of general anesthesia, shorter hospital stay, and the ability to manage symptoms at home.
- Up to half of patients with IPCs undergo spontaneous pleurodesis with resolution of their pleural effusion.

INTRODUCTION

Chronic recurrent pleural effusions provide a substantial disease burden in the United States, with 150,000 new malignant pleural effusions diagnosed each year.[1] Malignant pleural effusions have a particularly poor prognosis, with a mean life expectancy of approximately 4 months.[2] Because of the advanced disease state associated with these types of effusions, treatment is usually aimed at being palliative rather than curative. Therefore there is a particular focus on relief of symptoms, minimizing discomfort, minimizing disruption of daily life, and cost effectiveness.[3,4]

The treatment of pleural effusions is based on symptoms.[5,6] Dyspnea is the most common symptom, followed by cough and chest discomfort.[3] Twenty-five percent of pleural effusions are asymptomatic,[7] often discovered incidentally on chest radiography. These patients do not receive any intervention until they become symptomatic.

CONSIDERATIONS FOR INDWELLING PLEURAL CATHETERS

There are many management options for chronic recurrent pleural effusions, which include observation, thoracentesis, temporary pleural catheter, tunneled permanent pleural catheter, pleurodesis via pleural catheter, video-assisted thoracic surgery (VATS) or open pleurodesis, VATS or open pleurectomy, and pleuroperitoneal shunt. This article focuses on tunneled permanent pleural catheters, also commonly referred to as indwelling pleural catheters (IPCs).

It has become accepted practice to use IPCs in the management of malignant pleural effusions; therefore, most of the following information is

The authors have nothing to disclose.
[a] Department of Surgery, University of Virginia Health System, 725-2B Walker Square, Charlottesville, VA 22903, USA; [b] Division of Thoracic and Cardiovascular Surgery, Department of Surgery, University of Virginia Health System, PO Box 800679, Charlottesville, VA 22908-0679, USA
* Corresponding author.
E-mail address: CLL2Y@hscmail.mcc.virginia.edu

based on this subset of patients. However, there is a growing acceptance for the use of IPCs in the treatment of nonmalignant recurrent pleural effusions as well.[8]

When determining whether a patient is a good candidate for an IPC, there are several factors that must be considered (**Box 1**)[4,5]:

- Symptoms: If the patient has a pleural effusion but is asymptomatic, it is common practice to refrain from intervening.
- How fast the effusion recurs: Pleural effusions that take more than 1 month to recur are typically managed with serial thoracenteses. Effusions that recur less than 1 month after initial thoracentesis are managed with a more invasive approach such as IPC or pleurodesis.
- Life expectancy of the patient: In patients with a short life expectancy (less than 3 months), there is an emphasis on minimizing the time they spend in hospital in their remaining days. Therefore, a procedure such as an IPC that allows for same-day discharge is favorable to a more invasive procedure that requires several days stay as an inpatient.
- Performance status/surgical candidacy: Again, there is an effort to avoid performing invasive procedures that would require a prolonged recovery period in patients who have a poor performance status or who have a short life expectancy.
- Trapped lung or endobronchial obstruction by tumor: Both of these scenarios are contraindications to chemical pleurodesis. Because the affected lung will never fully reexpand, the pleural surfaces will not appose and the pleural space will not be obliterated, leaving space for the effusion to recur.[5,9,10]
- Response to systemic therapy: Tumors causing pleural effusions that are more susceptible to systemic chemotherapy, such as lymphoma or breast cancer, have a longer life expectancy and more favorable prognosis, which should be factored into management decisions.
- Patient preference: Patients have varying levels of aversion to living with a catheter in their chest and managing this catheter at home. Those averse to catheters will favor an option such as pleurodesis.

ALTERNATIVES

Common alternatives to IPCs include serial thoracenteses and chemical pleurodesis. Serial thoracenteses are a good option for patients with a short life expectancy and pleural effusions that are slow to re-accumulate. However, it is not without its drawbacks, as each thoracentesis carries a risk of pneumothorax, infection, bleeding, creating loculations, as well as the discomfort associated with each needle stick and drainage.

In patients with quickly accumulating effusions, chemical pleurodesis is often considered to be the first-line therapy over IPCs. Talc is the most commonly used agent, followed by tetracycline and doxycycline. The main advantage of chemical pleurodesis is that it is fairly effective at resolving the pleural effusion in one procedure. Disadvantages include its more invasive nature, a median postprocedure hospital stay of 4 to 7 days, and a 20% to 30% failure rate.[11,12] There is also a low but potentially serious risk of experiencing an adult respiratory distress syndrome–type reaction after the procedure.[13,14]

ADVANTAGES AND DISADVANTAGES OF IPCS

Compared with the alternatives, IPCs offer several advantages (**Box 2**).[15]

In addition, up to half of these patients show spontaneous pleurodesis with the catheter in place, allowing for removal of the catheter once

---

| Box 1 |
| **Considerations before placing an IPC** |

- Symptoms
- How fast the effusion recurs
- Life expectancy of the patient
- Performance status/surgical candidacy
- Trapped lung or endobronchial obstruction by tumor
- Response to systemic therapy
- Patient preference

| Box 2 |
| **Advantages of IPCs** |

- No general anesthesia required
- Minimally invasive
- Shorter hospital stay (compared with pleurodesis)
- Only one procedure
- Long-term control
- Spontaneous pleurodesis in up to half of patients

the output becomes sufficiently low.[16] The catheter causes an inflammatory reaction as it moves over the pleura with the respiratory cycle, leading to adhesions and apposition of the visceral and parietal pleura.[15]

The main disadvantages are listed in **Box 3**.

Recently there has been debate on the cost effectiveness of the various options for treating chronic recurrent pleural effusions. IPCs appear to be more cost effective, particularly for patients with short life expectancies, because the procedure cost is lower than pleurodesis, the postprocedure stay is shorter, and these patients have fewer readmissions and repeat procedures.[5] However, one factor that mitigates the cost effectiveness of IPCs is the need for several disposable vacuum drainage containers each week.

Two recent articles have attempted to address this question of cost effectiveness. An analysis by Olden and Holloway[17] using an estimated survival time of 6 months concluded that talc pleurodesis was more cost effective than IPCs, ($8170 vs $9011). An analysis by Puri and colleagues[18] reached a different conclusion. When using an estimated survival time of 3 months, they calculated the cost to be lowest with repeat thoracentesis ($4946), followed by IPC ($6450), bedside pleurodesis ($11,224), and thoracoscopic pleurodesis ($18,604). When performing the same calculations using an estimated survival time of 12 months, IPC and bedside pleurodesis were both similar in cost, at about $13,000.

Traditionally chemical pleurodesis has been the first-line treatment for chronic recurrent pleural effusions. However, IPCs have slowly gained more acceptance in this patient population. Many clinicians consider that IPCs are a superior first-line treatment for malignant pleural effusions because of their shorter postprocedure hospital stay, less frequent hospital admissions, and close to 50% rate of spontaneous pleurodesis.[3,19]

The authors use both chemical pleurodesis and IPCs as first-line treatment for chronic recurrent pleural effusions (**Fig. 1**). This decision is based on life expectancy, the patient's ability to tolerate general anesthesia, and patient preference. If a chemical pleurodesis is performed and the lung does not expand, an IPC is placed. The possibility of failed pleurodesis and subsequent IPC placement is discussed with the patient before the operation.

TYPES OF CATHETERS

The first case report of a patient being sent home with an IPC was in 1986. A Tenckhoff catheter was placed in the patient's pleural space, with drainage of the pleural effusion twice a week at home to relieve his dyspnea related to fluid accumulation.[20] In 1987, a small case series was published of patients with chest tubes or Foley catheters placed in the pleural space and attached to a collection system. These patients were similarly sent home with instructions to intermittently drain their pleural space.[21]

Through the 1990s there was a slow increase in the use of permanent pleural catheters that patients could use to drain their pleural effusions at home. In 1997, the Food and Drug Administration approved the PleurX catheter made by Denver Biomedical for use as a permanent indwelling pleural catheter to intermittently drain chronic recurrent pleural effusions. Since this approval, use of IPCs has become standard practice in the care of chronic pleural effusions.

The PleurX catheter (Denver Biomedical Inc, Golden, CO) continues to be the industry standard for IPCs (**Fig. 2**). It is a 15.5F soft silicone catheter, 66 cm in length with side holes over the distal 24 cm. Proximal to the side holes is a polyester cuff that is positioned just deep to the level of the skin to prevent the incidence of infection as well as inadvertent catheter dislodgment. The catheter also has a one-way safety valve that allows fluid to be drained out of the pleural space while also keeping fluid and air from entering into the pleural space. Vacuum bottles are hooked to the catheter to drain the pleural fluid. The system has recently been modified to prevent easy dislodgment when connected to a chest-tube drainage device.

The primary competitor in the United States is the Aspira pleural drainage system made by Bard Access Systems (Salt Lake City, UT). Its design is very similar to that of the PleurX. The primary difference is that instead of using vacuum bottles for pleural drainage, the Aspira catheter uses a manual pump (**Fig. 3**). The catheter is attached to a collection bag with the pump in line. The patient squeezes the pump to initiate the vacuum effect and the pleural fluid then drains into the collection bag.

The other primary catheter manufacturer is Rocket Medical in the United Kingdom. Again,

---

Box 3
Disadvantages of IPCs

- Lower pleurodesis rate/effusion resolution rate compared with chemical pleurodesis
- Risk of catheter-related infection
- Need for home support for catheter management

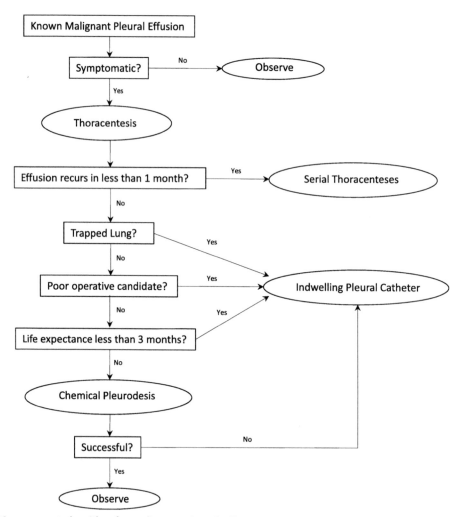

Fig. 1. Management algorithm for malignant pleural effusions.

their design is very similar to that of the PleurX catheter, with a 16F soft silicone catheter, 40 cm in length with side holes over the distal 24 cm.

PLACEMENT OF CATHETER

Placement of IPCs is routinely an outpatient procedure,[22] unless the patient is already admitted for another reason. The authors provide patients with teaching videos developed by the catheter manufacturer prior to their IPC placement so they can be more familiar and better prepared for handling these catheters.

The patient is positioned supine with a small roll (or Roho) under the side and the axilla on the side of the pleural effusion exposed. The patient is usually given conscious sedation during the procedure. The chest is prepped and draped in the usual sterile fashion. Local anesthetic is used at the puncture site as well as through the course

of the planned subcutaneous tunnel. Typically, ultrasound is used to visualize the pleural fluid and determine a safe window for catheter placement.[5] An 18- or 21-gauge needle is inserted through the skin in the mid to posterior axillary line, guided over the rib through the intercostal space and into the pleural space. The angle of the needle is directed posterior toward the posterior costophrenic sulcus. The wire is fed through the needle into the pleural space, and the needle is removed over the wire. A 1-cm incision is made at the guide-wire site, and a 1- to 2-cm incision is made at the chosen exit site for the catheter, approximately 5 cm anterior and inferior to the guide wire. Next, a subcutaneous tunnel is created between the 2 sites and the catheter is pulled through the tunnel until the cuff is just under the skin. A 16F peel-away introducer sheath is passed over the wire into the pleural space. It is important that the wire be movable at all times

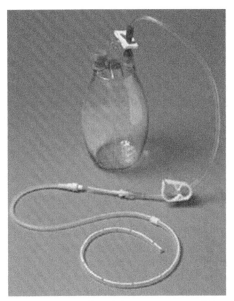

Fig. 2. The PleurX catheter drainage system. (*Courtesy of* CareFusion Corp, San Diego, CA; with permission.)

within the introducer to ensure proper placement of the introducer. The wire is removed and the catheter is fed through the sheath. The sheath is then peeled away, leaving the catheter within the pleural space. At this point, care is taken to make sure the catheter lies flat within the subcutaneous tunnel without any kinks. The skin is closed at the puncture site and the catheter is secured to the skin. This stitch is typically removed after

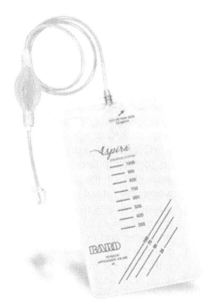

Fig. 3. The Aspira catheter drainage system. (*Courtesy of* Bard Access Systems, Salt Lake City, UT; © 2012 C. R. Bard, Inc. Used with permission.)

2 weeks once the catheter cuff has been secured with scar tissue.

MANAGEMENT OF CATHETER AFTER PLACEMENT

After catheter placement in the operating room or clinic, the tubing is generally initially hooked up to a chest-tube drainage device to allow drainage of the pleural effusion and to ensure no air leak is present from the procedure. The kit used generally has an adapter that easily allows this connection to be performed. General practice is to remove up to 1500 mL during this initial drainage session. With removal of greater than 1500 mL, the patient is at increased risk of experiencing reexpansion pulmonary edema, which can be life threatening.[5] If the patient begins experiencing chest tightness or pain, the catheter is disconnected and the cap is placed on the catheter. This pain is often due to the negative pressure created in the pleural space with removal of the pleural fluid,[23] often in the setting of a trapped lung that is struggling to reexpand fully. After a standard radiograph the authors usually cap the catheter if the effusion is drained, the lung is reexpanded, and there is no air leak present.

The key advantage of IPCs is that they allow for drainage and management of recurrent pleural effusions without a visit to the hospital. Therefore, after catheter placement, the patient and patient's family are taught how to use and care for the catheter at home. If the patient and family are not able to manage the catheter independently, visits from a home health nurse may be arranged.

There are several elements included in catheter education for the patient (**Box 4**). Patients are instructed on sterile technique when handling

---

Box 4
Home management tips

- Drain pleural fluid using sterile technique every 1 to 2 days
- Do not drain more than 1000 mL in one session
- Keep the catheter exit site dressed with sterile dressing
- Patient may shower if exit site is covered with a watertight dressing
- No bathing or swimming
- Monitor for signs of infection
- If less than 50 mL is removed on 3 consecutive drainings, one may consider removing catheter

the catheter tip. When not being used, the tip is covered with a cap to maintain sterility. For drainage of pleural fluid, the catheter cover is removed and the catheter is connected to the drainage bottle or drainage bag tubing. After drainage, the tubing is disconnected, the catheter tip is cleaned, and the cap is replaced. The patient is also instructed on how to clean and dress the skin exit site of the catheter.

The patient may shower or sponge-bathe if the catheter is covered with a watertight dressing. If the dressing gauze gets wet, the patient should change the dressing. Bathing, swimming, or any other activity that submerges the catheter entry site under water is prohibited.

Normally, patients are instructed to drain their pleural space either once a day or once every 2 days. Patients should not drain more than 1000 mL of fluid during one session at home, again to prevent reexpansion pulmonary edema.[7] Patients may complain of some chest pain with the initial drainage sessions, which is often due to the visceral and parietal pleura reapproximating with the catheter in between irritating the pleura.[5,7] Drainage is continued at home every 1 or 2 days until less than 50 mL is removed 3 sessions in a row. At this point the patient has likely undergone pleurodesis, and he or she is instructed to make an appointment with the physician for possible catheter removal. A chest radiograph is performed at the visit to confirm complete drainage of the pleural effusion before catheter removal.

Patient education also includes discussion of possible catheter complications. Patients are instructed on signs and symptoms of catheter infection: pain, redness, and swelling at the catheter site, change in character of pleural fluid, and fevers. If the catheter tubing is accidentally cut, patients are instructed to clamp the tubing proximal to the cut to prevent entry of air into the pleural space, and to call their physician. The catheter kit comes with a clamp for this particular situation.

Continued follow-up and monitoring after catheter placement is crucial for safety and effectiveness.[19] Physicians inserting these catheters must be committed to its ongoing care, akin to peritoneal dialysis catheters. IPCs are placed by physicians in several different specialties, and there is often no centralized follow-up for these patients. For these reasons, a dedicated IPC service at a given hospital is recommended.

IPC OUTCOMES

As the use of IPCs for management of malignant pleural effusions has increased over the past 15 years, there has been a growing body of data regarding their safety and effectiveness. There have been several case series of IPCs used to manage malignant pleural effusions, the largest published by Tremblay in 2006 (223 patients), Warren in 2008 (202 patients), and Suzuki in 2011 (355 patients).[15,24,25] In general, well over 90% of patients experience symptomatic improvement after IPC placement.[24,26] Approximately 90% of patients require no further procedures for the management of their pleural effusion after IPC placement.[24,25] In addition, the rate of spontaneous pleurodesis in IPC patients has been reported to be between 26% and 58%.[11,15,24,25]

The first randomized controlled trial comparing IPCs with chemical pleurodesis was conducted in 1999 by Putnam and colleagues,[27] who compared 91 patients who received an IPC for their malignant pleural effusion with 28 patients who instead underwent doxycycline pleurodesis via tube thoracostomy. The investigators found similar rates of survival, effusion recurrence, and adverse events between the 2 study groups. However, there was a significantly shorter hospitalization time in the IPC group (1 day vs 6.5 days).

More recently, there have been several nonrandomized trials comparing IPCs with talc pleurodesis. Two of the larger and most recent were performed by the groups of Hunt and Fysh in 2012.[28,29] Both studies demonstrated shorter length of hospital stay and fewer pleural reinterventions in the IPC patients compared with pleurodesis patients. These studies argue for a better quality of life, reduced disruption of life, and lower health care costs with IPCs.

In the June 2012 issue of the *Journal of the American Medical Association*, Davies and colleagues[11] published their randomized controlled trial comparing IPCs with talc pleurodesis via chest tube. A total of 106 patients who had not previously undergone pleurodesis were enrolled in the study. There was a significantly shorter length of stay after the procedure for the IPC group (0 days vs 4 days). More of the IPC patients experienced adverse events related to their procedure, but many of these were episodes of the catheter becoming clogged. However, the rate of repeat interventions on the pleural space was significantly higher in the pleurodesis group (22% vs 6%).

In 2011, van Meter and colleagues[16] compiled the most comprehensive review to date of outcomes for IPCs in the treatment of malignant pleural effusions. On analysis of data from 19 studies (1 randomized controlled trial, 18 case series) totaling 1370 patients, they found that 96% of patients showed improvement in symptoms, 46% of patients reached spontaneous pleurodesis with subsequent catheter removal, and 88% of patients had no complications related to the pleural catheter. Among the complications, the most frequent were symptomatic loculations (8%), empyema (3.8%), superficial cellulitis (3.4%), and clogged catheter (3.7%).

There are also increasing reports of the effectiveness of IPCs in the management of chronic nonmalignant pleural effusions. The groups of Parsaei and Borgeson[30,31] have both presented abstracts of their case series of patients with benign pleural effusions who were managed with IPCs. Together they found a 58% to 64% spontaneous pleurodesis rate, and an 8% to 16% infection rate. Borgeson and colleagues[31] also demonstrated a reduced rate of hospitalization at 6 and 12 months in IPC patients compared with their rate of hospitalization before IPC placement.

Chalhoub and colleagues[8] published their own case series of patients with malignant and nonmalignant pleural effusions who received an IPC. In their study, patients with nonmalignant pleural effusions took longer to reach spontaneous pleurodesis (111 days vs 36 days), but surprisingly all of their study patients did reach spontaneous pleurodesis. Because of the longer time to spontaneous pleurodesis, there is a higher concern for the infection risk in patients with nonmalignant pleural effusions. However, this study, albeit small, showed only 1 case of superficial cellulitis in 23 patients, with no cases of empyema, in contrast to one of the early case series of 5 patients with benign pleural effusions due to congestive heart failure treated with IPC, of whom 2 developed empyema and 1 died of sepsis.[32] The other major concern in patients with nonmalignant pleural effusions is the loss of protein, electrolytes, and fluid via the pleural tube. In Chalhoub's study,[8] patients were instructed to remove no more than 500 mL of fluid at any time. With this parameter in place, none of these patients reported any episodes of hypotension or laboratory abnormalities with their IPCs in place.

CATHETER COMPLICATIONS

Although the literature demonstrates the relative safety and less invasive nature of IPCs, there are some complications associated with these catheters (**Box 5**). Possible complications at the time of catheter placement include pneumothorax and lung injury, both of which are rare, and postprocedure pain. Catheter placement is usually very well tolerated with patients typically able to be discharged to home the same day.

Delayed catheter complications include catheter-related infections (superficial cellulitis,

---

Box 5
Catheter complications

Early
- Pneumothorax
- Bleeding
- Lung injury
- Postprocedure pain

Late
- Infection
- Catheter lumen obstruction
- Symptomatic loculations
- Accidental catheter removal

---

empyema), obstruction of the catheter lumen with debris, symptomatic loculations, and accidental removal of catheter. There have also been reported incidents of metastases along the catheter tract, which may be unsettling to the patient.[33] These metastases are typically treated effectively with radiation therapy.

Another uncommon late complication is fracture or iatrogenic severing of the IPC. Fysh and colleagues[34] reported a series of 6 patients with this complication noted at the time of patient presentation for catheter removal. In the 6 patients, either a catheter fracture was noted at the time of catheter removal or the catheter was so scarred into the pleural space that it could not be removed and was therefore cut and allowed to retract into the pleural space. Four patients retained catheter fragments in their pleural space, none of whom experienced any complications related to pain or infection as of the time of publication. Of note, all patients in this series had catheters made by Rocket Medical. There have been no reported cases in the literature of catheter fracture in PleurX or Aspira catheters.

Casal and colleagues[35] made a rather astute observation of complications in the spring of 2008. These investigators began noticing a relatively high incidence of PleurX catheter complications, including accidental dislodgments, pleural fluid leakage around the catheter site, and catheter site infections. When removing the PleurX catheters, they also noted a relative lack of fibrosis and scarring around the catheter cuff. Casal and colleagues hypothesized that a change in cuff manufacturing was the culprit, a suspicion that was validated after speaking with the catheter manufacturer. December 2007 through March 2008 was identified as the period when catheters with defective cuffs may have been distributed. On comparing complication rates in this group with the rates in IPC patients before and after this period, the investigators found an increased rate of complications (43% vs 13%), infections (15% vs 3%), and accidental dislodgments (11% vs 1%) in the study group.

SUMMARY

Tunneled IPCs have been a welcome addition to the treatment of chronic recurrent pleural effusions. These catheters offer a less invasive procedure with a short postprocedure hospital stay as well as a low incidence of repeat hospitalizations for effusion-related complications. IPCs also allow the patient greater control of their symptoms, with the ability to manage their symptoms at home. Further randomized controlled studies are needed to more clearly differentiate which patients are best served by an IPC as their initial intervention, rather than traditional pleurodesis.

REFERENCES

1. Antony VB, Loddenkemper R, Astoul P, et al. Management of malignant pleural effusions. Eur Respir J 2001;18(2):402–19.
2. Burrows CM, Mathews WC, Colt HG. Predicting survival in patients with recurrent symptomatic malignant pleural effusions: an assessment of the prognostic values of physiologic, morphologic, and quality of life measures of extent of disease. Chest 2000;117(1):73–8.
3. Pollak JS. Malignant pleural effusions: treatment with tunneled long-term drainage catheters. Curr Opin Pulm Med 2002;8(4):302–7.
4. Kaifi JT, Toth JW, Gusani NJ, et al. Multidisciplinary management of malignant pleural effusion. J Surg Oncol 2012;105(7):731–8.
5. Roberts ME, Neville E, Berrisford RG, et al. Management of a malignant pleural effusion: British Thoracic Society Pleural Disease Guideline 2010. Thorax 2010;65(Suppl 2):ii32–40.
6. Antunes G, Neville E. Management of malignant pleural effusions. Thorax 2000;55(12):981–3.
7. Spector M, Pollak JS. Management of malignant pleural effusions. Semin Respir Crit Care Med 2008;29(4):405–13.
8. Chalhoub M, Harris K, Castellano M, et al. The use of the PleurX catheter in the management of non-malignant pleural effusions. Chron Respir Dis 2011;8(3):185–91.
9. Pien GW, Gant MJ, Washam CL, et al. Use of an implantable pleural catheter for trapped lung syndrome in patients with malignant pleural effusion. Chest 2001;119(6):1641–6.
10. Qureshi RA, Collinson SL, Powell RJ, et al. Management of malignant pleural effusion associated with trapped lung syndrome. Asian Cardiovasc Thorac Ann 2008;16(2):120–3.
11. Davies HE, Mishra EK, Kahan BC, et al. Effect of an indwelling pleural catheter vs chest tube and talc pleurodesis for relieving dyspnea in patients with malignant pleural effusion: the TIME2 randomized controlled trial. JAMA 2012;307(22):2383–9.
12. Dresler CM, Olak J, Herndon JE 2nd, et al. Phase III intergroup study of talc poudrage vs talc slurry sclerosis for malignant pleural effusion. Chest 2005;127(3):909–15.
13. Thompson RL, Yau JC, Donnelly RF, et al. Pleurodesis with iodized talc for malignant effusions using pigtail catheters. Ann Pharmacother 1998;32(7–8):739–42.
14. Rehse DH, Aye RW, Florence MG. Respiratory failure following talc pleurodesis. Am J Surg 1999;177(5):437–40.
15. Warren WH, Kalimi R, Khodadadian LM, et al. Management of malignant pleural effusions using the Pleur(x) catheter. Ann Thorac Surg 2008;85(3):1049–55.
16. Van Meter ME, McKee KY, Kohlwes RJ. Efficacy and safety of tunneled pleural catheters in adults with malignant pleural effusions: a systematic review. J Gen Intern Med 2011;26(1):70–6.
17. Olden AM, Holloway R. Treatment of malignant pleural effusion: PleuRx catheter or talc pleurodesis? A cost-effectiveness analysis. J Palliat Med 2010;13(1):59–65.
18. Puri V, Pyrdeck TL, Crabtree TD, et al. Treatment of malignant pleural effusion: a cost-effectiveness analysis. Ann Thorac Surg 2012;94(2):374–9.
19. Lee YC, Fysh ET. Indwelling pleural catheter: changing the paradigm of malignant effusion management. J Thorac Oncol 2011;6(4):655–7.
20. Leff RS, Eisenberg B, Baisden CE, et al. Drainage of recurrent pleural effusion via an implanted port and intrapleural catheter. Ann Intern Med 1986;104(2):208–9.
21. Hewitt JB, Janssen WR. A management strategy for malignancy-induced pleural effusion: long-term thoracostomy drainage. Oncol Nurs Forum 1987;14(5):17–22.
22. Pollak JS, Burdge CM, Rosenblatt M, et al. Treatment of malignant pleural effusions with tunneled long-term drainage catheters. J Vasc Interv Radiol 2001;12(2):201–8.
23. Feller-Kopman D, Walkey A, Berkowitz D, et al. The relationship of pleural pressure to symptom development during therapeutic thoracentesis. Chest 2006;129(6):1556–60.
24. Tremblay A, Michaud G. Single-center experience with 250 tunnelled pleural catheter insertions for malignant pleural effusion. Chest 2006;129(2):362–8.

25. Suzuki K, Servais EL, Rizk NP, et al. Palliation and pleurodesis in malignant pleural effusion: the role for tunneled pleural catheters. J Thorac Oncol 2011;6(4):762–7.

26. Chen YM, Shih JF, Yang KY, et al. Usefulness of pig-tail catheter for palliative drainage of malignant pleural effusions in cancer patients. Support Care Cancer 2000;8(5):423–6.

27. Putnam JB Jr, Light RW, Rodriguez RM, et al. A randomized comparison of indwelling pleural catheter and doxycycline pleurodesis in the management of malignant pleural effusions. Cancer 1999;86(10):1992–9.

28. Fysh ET, Waterer GW, Kendall P, et al. Indwelling pleural catheters reduce inpatient days over pleurodesis for malignant pleural effusion. Chest 2012;142(2):394–400.

29. Hunt BM, Farivar AS, Vallieres E, et al. Thoracoscopic talc versus tunneled pleural catheters for palliation of malignant pleural effusions. Ann Thorac Surg 2012;94(4):1053–9.

30. Parsaei N, Khodaverdian R, Mckelvey AA, et al. Use of long-term indwelling tunneled pleural catheter for the management of benign pleural effusion. Chest 2006;130(Suppl):271S.

31. Borgeson DD, Defranchi SA, Lam CS, et al. Chronic indwelling pleural catheters reduce hospitalizations in advanced heart failure with refractory pleural effusions. J Card Fail 2009;15(Suppl):105S.

32. Herlihy JP, Loyalka P, Gnananandh J, et al. PleurX catheter for the management of refractory pleural effusions in congestive heart failure. Tex Heart Inst J 2009;36(1):38–43.

33. Janes SM, Rahman NM, Davies RJ, et al. Catheter-tract metastases associated with chronic indwelling pleural catheters. Chest 2007;131(4):1232–4.

34. Fysh ET, Wrightson JM, Lee YC, et al. Fractured indwelling pleural catheters. Chest 2012;141(4):1090–4.

35. Casal RF, Bashoura L, Ost D, et al. Detecting medical device complications: lessons from an indwelling pleural catheter clinic. Am J Med Qual 2012. [Epub ahead of print].

Surgical Management of Malignant Pleural Mesothelioma

Jane Yanagawa, MD, Valerie Rusch, MD*

KEYWORDS

- Malignant pleural mesothelioma • Asbestos • Multimodality therapy • Extrapleural pneumonectomy
- Pleurectomy/decortication

KEY POINTS

- The incidence of malignant pleural mesothelioma is still increasing on a worldwide level despite the institution of regulations to minimize asbestos exposure, owing to its long latency period.
- Multimodality therapy (surgery, radiation therapy, and chemotherapy) provides the best results, although median survival is still poor (17–30 months).
- Whether to perform extrapleural pneumonectomy or pleurectomy/decortication is a controversial subject. The decision is frequently made in the operating room. Important considerations include the ability to achieve complete resection, the available adjuvant therapies, and the prognostic factors related to the individual and the tumor.

INTRODUCTION

Although malignant pleural mesothelioma (MPM) is a relatively uncommon disease, there is heightened awareness of it among the general public owing to its association with asbestos exposure and the resultant societal implications. Asbestos was commonly used in construction and manufacturing activities during most of the twentieth century. As the role of asbestos in the development of MPM became clear, the Occupational Safety and Health Administration and the Environmental Protection Agency instituted regulations to limit occupational exposure, beginning with the establishment of a permissible exposure limit for asbestos in 1971. Despite the sharp decline in asbestos exposure during the last few decades, approximately 2000 to 3000 cases are still diagnosed each year in the United States. Owing to the long latency period of 20 to 50 years for MPM, the incidence of MPM from decades-old exposures has yet to peak. In addition, new exposures continue to pose a threat.[1] Although asbestos is no longer mined in the United States, the mineral is still imported. Workers and surrounding communities are also at risk of new exposures if there are insufficient controls in place during the remediation and demolition of buildings with existing asbestos. The destruction of the World Trade Center towers during the tragedy on September 11, 2001 is an example of such a risk. MPM is far from being a historical disease; therefore, it is important for thoracic surgeons to understand how to manage patients who present with a possible diagnosis of MPM.

CLINICAL PRESENTATION

The clinical presentation of MPM is often nonspecific. In the early stages of the disease the most common presentation is dyspnea, usually associated with the presence of a pleural effusion. Drainage of the effusion may leave the patient

Thoracic Surgery Service, Department of Surgery, Memorial Sloan-Kettering Cancer Center, 1275 York Avenue, New York, NY 10065, USA
* Corresponding author.
E-mail address: ruschv@mskcc.org

Thorac Surg Clin 23 (2013) 73–87
http://dx.doi.org/10.1016/j.thorsurg.2012.10.002

asymptomatic. As the disease progresses, the patient may develop chest discomfort. Shortness of breath can improve if tumor progression leads to fusion of the pleural space, preventing the recurrence of pleural effusions. When the disease advances to the point of tumor infiltration into the chest wall or intercostal nerves, the patient may complain of unremitting chest pain. In such late stages of disease dyspnea becomes a problem again, secondary to encasement of the lung, mediastinum, and chest wall, at times compromising the function of the contralateral lung. The disease may spread through the diaphragm, causing ascites, or to the contralateral side, resulting in a contralateral pleural effusion.

Obtaining a thorough history includes performing a detailed investigation of the patient's exposure to asbestos. The Centers for Disease Control and Prevention National Institute for Occupational Safety and Health examined industry and occupation data for mesothelioma deaths that occurred in 1999 and found significant associations with industry involving ship and boat building and repair, industrial and miscellaneous chemicals, petroleum refining, electric light and power, and construction. Occupations at significant risk included plumbers, pipefitters, steamfitters, mechanical engineers, electricians, and elementary school teachers (**Box 1**).[2]

Relevant physical-examination findings during the early stages of disease are mainly those associated with pleural effusions. In later stages of disease, when the tumor encases the hemithorax, the chest wall may be contracted and include excursion of the chest, with respiration noticeably diminished. Diffuse dullness to percussion and decreased lung sounds may be present, in addition to a fullness of the intercostal spaces. Palpable soft-tissue masses may be present at previous biopsy sites or where the tumor has penetrated the chest wall. Supraclavicular or axillary lymphadenopathy or ascites may be present in metastatic disease.

Although uncommon, paraneoplastic syndromes may cause abnormalities in laboratory values, including autoimmune hemolytic anemia, hypercalcemia, hypoglycemia, the syndrome of inappropriate antidiuretic hormone, and thrombocytosis.

DIAGNOSIS

If a patient's clinical presentation is suggestive of MPM, the focus next turns to obtaining tissue for diagnosis. As most MPM patients present with pleural effusions, thoracentesis is frequently the first diagnostic procedure performed. Cytologic analysis of pleural fluid, however, identifies malignancy in only approximately 60% of cases. The yield from needle biopsy is better, at 86%, but cannot compete with the results of sampling from thoracoscopy, which is diagnostic for 98% of patients.[3,4] Thoracoscopy allows for biopsy of parietal, visceral, and diaphragmatic pleura, while remaining minimally invasive. Findings on thoracoscopy depend on the stage of disease: from a pleural effusion, to tumor studding of the parietal pleura only, to involvement of both the parietal and visceral pleura. More advanced disease may present as discrete tumor masses or sheets of tumor. If the pleural space has been obliterated by locally advanced tumor, making thoracoscopy impossible, the small incision created for thoracoscopy may be extended to 6 cm and the associated rib resected to allow for open pleural biopsy. As MPM has a tendency to implant in the chest wall at biopsy sites, incisions should always be strategically in line with potential future thoracotomy incisions, so that the scar can be excised at the time of surgery. To save patients with metastatic adenocarcinoma from unnecessary morbidity and to avoid further complicating the definitive surgical resection in patients who do have MPM, exploratory thoracotomy should not be performed before tissue diagnosis is obtained.

The histologic diagnosis of MPM can be difficult. MPMs are classified as epithelioid, sarcomatoid, biphasic (mixed epithelioid/sarcomatoid), or desmoplastic neoplasms. Epithelioid is the most common (>50%), biphasic is of intermediate

---

Box 1
Industries and occupations associated with asbestos exposure

Industries

Ship and boat building and repair

Industrial chemicals

Petroleum refining

Electric light and power

Construction

Occupations

Plumbers

Pipefitters

Steamfitters

Mechanical engineers

Electricians

Automotive workers

School teachers

frequency, sarcomatoid is less common (approximately 15%), and the desmoplastic form is very rare. To avoid misdiagnosis (epithelioid vs metastatic adenocarcinoma, sarcomatoid vs sarcoma, desmoplastic vs benign fibrosis), histochemical analysis and immunostaining play an important role in distinguishing MPMs from other tumors (**Table 1**). If the diagnosis remains in question after immunohistochemical analysis, electron microscopy can provide definitive results, although this is now rarely necessary. As the histologic subtype contributes not only to prognosis but also to surgical decision making, accurate diagnosis is critical.

STAGING AND PROGNOSTIC FACTORS

Defining a staging system for MPM was previously complicated by limitations in the understanding of the prognostic factors and the natural history of this relatively uncommon disease. In 1994, the International Mesothelioma Interest Group (IMIG) gathered a panel of international experts to develop the TNM-based system that is now available in the American Joint Commission on Cancer (AJCC) and the International Union Against Cancer (UICC) staging systems (**Table 2**). In this staging system, the regional lymph node (N) and distant metastasis (M) descriptions are similar to those for lung cancer staging, but the primary tumor (T) descriptors are markedly different, owing to the uniquely diffuse nature of the disease. T1a and T1b describe involvement of the ipsilateral parietal and visceral pleura, respectively. T2 disease involves the additional invasion of lung parenchyma or diaphragmatic muscle. T3 describes locally advanced but still potentially resectable

disease, whereas T4 describes locally advanced but technically unresectable disease.

In 1995, Rusch and Venkatraman[5] applied the new IMIG staging system to 131 patients who had been surgically treated for MPM and found statistically significant survival differences based on stage (median survival: stage I, 35 months; stage II, 16 months; stage III, 11.5 months; stage IV, 5.9 months), thereby validating the utility of this staging system for the identification of patients with poor prognosis. More recent studies suggest possible revisions to further enhance the predictive power of this staging system. For example, Flores and colleagues[6] evaluated 348 patients with surgically resected MPM and found that survival was influenced by the number of involved N2 stations (0, 1, 2, or more; $P<.01$), suggesting that disease with involvement of multiple N2 nodal sites could potentially be classified as higher stage than disease with single-station N2 involvement.

In addition to stage, histologic subtype is a well-established prognostic factor. Many thoracic surgeons do not operate on patients whose preoperative histologic analysis reveals the sarcomatoid subtype, as prognosis has been shown to be poor (median survival, 15.1 months for epithelioid vs 6 months for nonepithelioid).[5]

Imaging studies have introduced new ways to assess clinical T category and prognosis. Pass and colleagues[7] showed that, in the preoperative assessment of tumor volume, the results of volumetric computed tomography (CT) image analysis correlated with postoperative determinations of both T and N status and could predict overall and progression-free survival of patients undergoing cytoreductive surgery. These investigators also showed that residual postoperative tumor burden significantly influenced overall survival (median survival, 9 months for residual tumor burden >9 mL vs 25 months for residual tumor burden <9 mL; $P = .0002$). Flores and colleagues[8] showed more recently that tumor standardized uptake value (SUV) calculations from preoperative positron emission tomography (PET) imaging could also predict poor prognosis (median survival, 9.7 months for SUV >10 vs 21 months for SUV <10; $P = .02$).

TREATMENT
Surgery

For patients who are candidates for palliation only, pleurodesis and PleurX catheter placement are effective surgical options. Surgical interventions for the curative treatment of MPM include extrapleural pneumonectomy (EPP) and pleurectomy/decortication (P/D). EPP involves the en bloc

---

Table 1
Immunohistochemical analysis to differentiate MPM from adenocarcinoma

Histologic Analysis/ Immunostaining	MPM	Adenocarcinoma
Mucicarmine	−	+
Periodic acid-Schiff	−	+
Calretinin	+	−
Carcinoembryonic antigen	−	+
Cytokeratin	+	−
LeuM-1	−	+
Vimentin	+	−
Thyroid transcription factor 1	−	+
E-cadherin	−	+

Table 2
American Joint Commission on Cancer/International Union Against Cancer international staging system for MPM

Primary Tumor (T)

TX	Primary tumor cannot be assessed
T0	No evidence of primary tumor
T1	Tumor involves ipsilateral parietal pleura, with or without focal involvement of visceral pleura
T1a	Tumor involves ipsilateral parietal pleura (mediastinal, diaphragmatic) pleura, with no involvement of the visceral pleura
T1b	Tumor involves ipsilateral parietal (mediastinal, diaphragmatic) pleura, with focal involvement of the visceral pleura
T2	Tumor involves any of the ipsilateral pleural surfaces with at least 1 of the following: Confluent visceral pleural tumor (including fissure) Invasion of diaphragmatic muscle Invasion of lung parenchyma
T3	Describes locally advanced but potentially resectable tumor Tumor involves any of the ipsilateral pleural surfaces with at least 1 of the following: Invasion of the endothoracic fascia Invasion into mediastinal fat Solitary focus of tumor invading the soft tissues of the chest wall Nontransmural involvement of the pericardium
T4	Describes locally advanced, technically unresectable tumor Tumor involves any of the ipsilateral pleural surfaces with at least 1 of the following: Diffuse or multifocal invasion of soft tissues of the chest wall Any involvement of rib Invasion through the diaphragm to the peritoneum Direct extension of any mediastinal organs Direct extension to the contralateral pleura Invasion into the spine Extension to the internal surface of the pericardium Pericardial effusion with positive cytology Invasion of the myocardium Invasion of the brachial plexus

Regional Lymph Nodes (N)

NX	Regional lymph nodes cannot be assessed
N0	No regional lymph node metastases
N1	Metastases in the ipsilateral bronchopulmonary and/or hilar lymph nodes
N2	Metastases in the subcarinal lymph nodes and/or the ipsilateral internal mammary or mediastinal lymph nodes
N3	Metastases in the contralateral mediastinal, contralateral internal mammary, or hilar lymph nodes, and/or the ipsilateral or contralateral supraclavicular or scalene lymph nodes

Distant Metastasis (M)

MX	Distant metastases cannot be assessed
M0	No distant metastasis
M1	Distant metastasis present

Stage Grouping

Stage I	T1	N0	M0
Stage IA	T1a	N0	M0
Stage IB	T1b	N0	M0
Stage II	T2	N0	M0
Stage III	T1, T2	N1	M0
	T1, T2	N2	
	T3	N0, N1, N2	
Stage IV	T4	Any N	M0
	Any T	N3	M0
	Any T	Any N	M1

resection of the affected lung and pleura, pericardium, and hemidiaphragm. P/D includes the en bloc resection of the affected pleura, and the pericardium and hemidiaphragm, as needed, but leaves the lung intact. The goal of each procedure is the same: to completely remove all macroscopic disease. However, each offers different advantages, and there still exist insufficient data to provide clear-cut guidelines regarding which operation should be performed for any individual patient. Although there is considerable controversy concerning this topic, the decision to perform one operation over the other depends on the ability to provide a complete resection, the requirements of planned adjuvant therapy, and the patient's prognosis.[9]

In the treatment of MPM, the benefit of surgery remains largely assumed, as there have been no randomized studies to prove that surgery improves survival. Treasure and colleagues,[10] in the Mesothelioma and Radical Surgery feasibility study, attempted to address this issue by assessing the clinical outcomes of patients randomly assigned to EPP or no EPP in the context of trimodal therapy. The trial demonstrated the difficulty of recruiting patients to such a study, as it took 3 years to randomly assign the 50 patients (EPP, n = 24; no EPP, n = 26) they had hoped to accrue in 1 year. There were not enough patients included in the study to allow for any definitive conclusions to be drawn regarding the effect of EPP on overall survival, although the investigators reported a longer median survival for the no-EPP group than for the EPP group (19.5 vs 14.4 months). This result was in the context of chemotherapy regimens that were not standardized and an operative mortality (18%) that was greater than that usually reported in other studies of multimodality therapy (0%–5%), making it even more difficult to judge the utility of EPP in the management of MPM on the basis of this trial.

Ultimately surgery is widely accepted to be necessary, as improved survival has been correlated with the degree of cytoreduction.[7] The controversy lies in the type of surgery required to achieve this goal. The advantages of EPP include, theoretically, a more complete cytoreduction and the ability to administer adjuvant high-dose radiation, as a result of having removed the lung parenchyma from the treatment field, overall yielding significantly better local control than with P/D (local recurrence, 33% vs 65%).[11] The advantage of P/D lies mainly in the lower rates of surgical morbidity and mortality associated with it. Mortality for EPP ranges from 4% to 15%, and that for P/D ranges from 1% to 5%. Morbidity is 23% for EPP, compared with 10.5% for P/D.[12]

Because it is necessary to balance the oncologic goals of maximal cytoreduction and optimization of adjuvant therapies with considerations for patient-related and tumor-related prognostic factors, the decision regarding which procedure to perform is frequently made in the operating room. P/D may be performed for earlier-stage disease, when there is minimal visceral involvement and when complete cytoreduction can conceivably be achieved without removal of the lung. EPP may be the choice for the patient with greater tumor burden whose disease is still completely resectable. Obviously the decision to perform one procedure over the other is clear when patients are physiologically unable to endure a pneumonectomy. For patients with poor prognostic factors, such as those with sarcomatoid/mixed histology tumors (if these patients are to be considered for surgery at all) or positive mediastinal lymph node involvement (median survival, 10 months), P/D may be the best option, to spare these patients the increased risks associated with EPP. Of note, in a small retrospective study comparing outcomes of node-positive patients who underwent either EPP or P/D, Martin-Ucar and colleagues[13] found no survival difference between the 2 groups. Patients who are found to have unresectable disease on surgical exploration should undergo debulking to help minimize symptoms and maximize pulmonary reserve, to facilitate potential systemic therapy.

That there are clinical scenarios for which one operation is more likely than the other to be performed makes it difficult to directly compare the outcomes of the 2 procedures in retrospective studies. In 2008, Flores and colleagues[11] retrospectively reviewed 663 consecutive patients who underwent resection for MPM at 3 institutions between 1990 and 2006. The operative mortality was 7% for EPP and 4% for P/D. EPP was associated with worse survival compared with P/D (median survival, 12 vs 16 months; P<.001), but this was likely related to selection bias. The 2 groups were statistically significantly different in terms of age (60 vs 63 years), early stage (25% vs 35%), and multimodality therapy (69% vs 58%) for EPP versus P/D, and they were also likely different in ways that are not reflected in such easily measured characteristics.

Chemotherapy

MPM has historically been considered to be chemoresistant, as median survival was essentially no different between patients treated with supportive care (6–8 months) and those treated with single-agent chemotherapy (6–9 months).[14]

The introduction of platinum-based combination therapies has been associated with improved response rates, and the recent addition of antifolate agents has yielded results that solidify chemotherapy as an effective option in the treatment of MPM. The breakthrough study establishing the combination of cisplatin and pemetrexed (antifolate agent) as the first-line chemotherapy regimen for MPM was published in 2003 by Vogelzang and colleagues.[15] The article reported the results of a large (448 patients), multicenter, randomized phase III trial that compared cisplatin alone with cisplatin plus pemetrexed in patients with unresectable MPM. The investigators found a significantly improved median survival time (12.1 vs 9.3 months; $P = .02$) and a longer median time to disease progression (5.7 vs 3.9 months; $P = .001$) in the cisplatin plus pemetrexed group, compared with the cisplatin-alone group. The response rate was 41.3% versus 16.7% ($P<.001$) in favor of the combination-therapy group. These results have led to the use of this chemotherapy regimen in more recent trials of multimodality therapies.

Radiation Therapy

Mesothelioma cells are moderately radiosensitive, and the option of adjuvant radiation is particularly attractive because of the high local recurrence rate (80%) after surgical resection alone. However, the use of radiation therapy with curative intent is restricted by the injury incurred by the intact lung when radiation therapy is administered at therapeutic doses. Studies have shown that hemithoracic radiation at doses greater than 45 Gy can cause severe deterioration of pulmonary function that is equivalent to total loss of lung function on the irradiated side.[16] However, when hemithoracic radiation is administered after P/D (lung still in place) at low to moderate doses (20–45 Gy), there is both a lack of efficacy and significant toxicity. In addition, there is a high rate of locally recurrent disease (35%) when hemithoracic radiation is administered at low doses after EPP.[17,18] At Memorial Sloan-Kettering Cancer Center (MSKCC), it was hypothesized that higher doses of radiation should be tolerable after EPP, with the at-risk lung parenchyma removed. A phase II trial of 54 patients who underwent EPP followed by high-dose hemithoracic radiation (54 Gy) showed that this regimen of treatment was not only feasible but that, compared with historical controls, it dramatically reduced local recurrence (13%) and was associated with prolonged survival among patients with early-stage disease (median survival, 33.8 months).[19] At present, in the treatment of MPM the use of radiation therapy alone is recommended only for palliation of symptomatic localized tumors of the chest wall or mediastinum or for prevention of local recurrences after thoracentesis and thoracoscopic biopsy.[20]

Trimodality Therapy

Although the combination of EPP and adjuvant radiation has led to much-improved local control (as in the aforementioned phase II study), distant recurrence remained a problem in more than 60% of patients, and overall survival was only 10 months for patients with stage III and IV disease.[19] The addition of chemotherapy to the multimodality therapy aims to reduce the risk of systemic relapse and improve overall survival. Several trimodality studies, incorporating EPP, systemic chemotherapy, and external-beam radiation therapy, suggest that such treatment strategies improve survival (**Table 3**).[21–29]

The largest such prospective study to date (N = 77) was a multicenter phase II trial that tested the combination of induction pemetrexed plus cisplatin, followed by EPP and radiation therapy (54 Gy), for fit patients with early-stage (I–III) MPM.[27] Median survival was 16.8 months for the intention-to-treat group, 21.9 months for those who underwent EPP (74%), and 29.1 months for those who completed all 3 therapies (52%). Among the patients who underwent surgery, the distant relapse rate was 26%, with total relapse-free rates of 63.8% at 1 year and 38.9% at 2 years. Of note, complete or partial response to chemotherapy was associated with a median survival nearly twice as long as that for patients who had stable or progressive disease (26 vs 13.9 months; $P = .05$). These results suggest that, for patients able to complete the multimodality regimen, trimodality therapy is feasible and provides reasonably long-term survival.

Achieving further improvements in overall survival will most likely rely on innovations in neoadjuvant and adjuvant therapies, but what influence the type of operation (EPP vs P/D) has on the results of trimodality therapy remains a question. In prospective studies of trimodality therapy that includes EPP, the percentage of patients who complete all therapies ranges from 33% to 63%.[30] The inclusion of P/D in a trimodality regimen is attractive because one would assume that a procedure with lower associated morbidity might result in more patients completing all therapies. Owing to the limitations of adjuvant radiation therapy after P/D, there are far fewer investigations of P/D with the traditional combination of chemotherapy and external-beam radiation therapy. In an attempt to improve local control, P/D has

Table 3
Prospective trials of trimodality therapy (surgery, chemotherapy, and adjuvant radiation) for MPM

Authors,[Ref.] Year	No. of Patients	Surgery	Radiation Therapy (Gy)	Chemotherapy	Median Survival (mo)	ITT to Complete All Therapy (%)
Weder et al,[21] 2004	19	EPP	30–60	Neoadjuvant gemcitabine/cisplatin	23	32
Pagan et al,[22] 2006	54	EPP	50	Adjuvant paclitaxel/carboplatin	20	57
Flores et al,[23] 2006	21	EPP	54	Neoadjuvant gemcitabine/cisplatin	19	33
Weder et al,[24] 2007	61	EPP	50–60	Neoadjuvant gemcitabine/cisplatin	20	39
Rea et al,[25] 2007	21	EPP	45	Neoadjuvant gemcitabine/carboplatin	25	62
Batirel et al,[26] 2008	20	EPP	54	Adjuvant gemcitabine/cisplatin or adjuvant pemetrexed/cisplatin	17	60
Krug et al,[27] 2009	77	EPP	54	Neoadjuvant pemetrexed/cisplatin	17	52
Bolukbas et al,[28] 2011	35	P/D	45–50	Adjuvant pemetrexed/cisplatin	30	94
Van Schil et al,[29] 2010	59	EPP	54	Neoadjuvant gemcitabine/cisplatin	18	63

Abbreviations: EPP, extrapleural pneumonectomy; ITT, intention to treat; P/D, pleurectomy/decortication.

been tested with a variety of intrapleural therapies, such as photodynamic therapy, intracavitary chemotherapy (with and without hyperthermia), brachytherapy, and intrapleural immunotherapeutic agents.[31–33] Although some of these strategies have been shown to be safe and feasible, few have resulted in significantly improved survival; such strategies, therefore, require further study.

A new approach to the problem of adjuvant therapy after P/D may lie in the development of more sophisticated radiation delivery techniques. In intensity-modulated radiation therapy (IMRT), the intensity of the radiation is modified, based on 3-dimensional treatment planning, to deliver more radiation to the tumor while sparing surrounding normal tissues. Although initial use after either EPP or P/D led to unacceptable pulmonary toxicity, adjustments have been made to IMRT delivery techniques that have resulted in fewer complications. In a retrospective study by Rosenzweig and colleagues,[34] 20 patients underwent IMRT to the pleura after P/D, with acceptable levels of morbidity observed. Median survival was 26 months. A phase II trial of neoadjuvant chemotherapy followed by P/D and IMRT to the pleura is currently under way at MSKCC.

CLINICAL GUIDELINES
Preoperative Evaluation

The main goal of the preoperative evaluation is to determine whether the patient is amenable to complete resection and whether the patient has the cardiopulmonary reserve to undergo EPP.

To identify patients who have either unresectable or metastatic disease, CT imaging of the chest and abdomen is routinely performed as initial staging studies. CT imaging is far better than standard radiography at demonstrating the extent of pleural disease, as well as mediastinal and pericardial involvement. CT imaging, however, is less effective for the diagnosis of chest-wall involvement and extension through the diaphragm. A prospective study comparing CT and magnetic resonance imaging (MRI) showed that neither imaging study was superior to the other in this regard.[35] On the other hand, ^{18}F-fluorodeoxyglucose (FDG)-PET contributes to staging through the identification of extrathoracic metastases. In an analysis of 60 preoperative PET studies, occult distant disease was identified in 10% of patients who had been deemed resectable by CT imaging.[36] Integrated PET/CT may be even more sensitive.[37] Bronchoscopy is unnecessary preoperatively, as MPM does not present as endobronchial disease. Preoperative diagnosis of nodal involvement remains difficult. Owing to the pattern of nodal metastases in MPM (lymphatic drainage from pleura to internal mammary, paravertebral, and peridiaphragmatic areas), mediastinoscopy fails to identify the majority of patients with N2 disease. However, routine mediastinoscopy/endobronchial ultrasonography and laparoscopy are invasive staging procedures advocated by some investigators for the identification of transdiaphragmatic invasion and nodal metastases.[38] At MSKCC surgeons/physicians perform MRI, nodal biopsies, and laparoscopy selectively, based on clinical findings and initial imaging studies.

The assessment of cardiopulmonary reserve begins with pulmonary function testing. This study should include a measurement of the carbon monoxide–diffusing capacity of the lung (D_{Lco}), as patients who have had exposure to asbestos frequently have a more dramatic decrease of D_{Lco} compared with forced expiratory volume at 1 second, because of their underlying interstitial lung disease. Exercise and resting arterial blood gases can provide a qualitative estimate of cardiopulmonary reserve. To calculate the pulmonary function after a potential EPP, a quantitative ventilation/perfusion lung scan should also be performed. Because many patients with MPM are older, with medical comorbidities, a thorough cardiovascular evaluation should be performed to determine the patient's risk for myocardial ischemia, as the operation may involve significant intraoperative blood loss and perioperative fluid shifts. At MSKCC, this evaluation includes a nuclear medicine stress echocardiogram (**Box 2**).

Box 2
Recommended preoperative workup for patients with MPM

Staging

CT chest and abdomen

PET/CT imaging

Physiologic Workup

Pulmonary function testing

Ventilation/perfusion scan

Nuclear medicine stress echocardiogram

Optional Evaluation

MRI chest and abdomen

Laparoscopy

Mediastinoscopy or endobronchial ultrasonography

Surgical Technique

The ultimate decision of whether to perform P/D or EPP is frequently made intraoperatively, and both dissections begin identically, allowing the potential to perform either procedure after the initial surgical exploration.

An epidural catheter is placed by the anesthesiologist for postoperative analgesia. After the induction of general anesthesia, a double-lumen endotracheal tube is inserted. Intraoperative monitoring should include arterial line, pulse oximetry, and a central line to allow for perioperative monitoring of central venous pressure.

The patient is then placed in the standard lateral decubitus position. An extended S-shaped posterolateral thoracotomy incision is made, with the inferior portion curving down to the costal margin (**Fig. 1**). This maneuver allows for adequate exposure for diaphragmatic resection and reconstruction. Previous biopsy incisions are incorporated into the thoracotomy or chest-tube sites, if possible. Latissimus dorsi and serratus anterior muscles are both divided. The sixth rib is excised to expose the extrapleural plane, with care taken to preserve the intercostal muscle for closure if an EPP is performed (**Fig. 2**). Blunt dissection is initiated in the extrapleural plane, between the parietal pleura and the endothoracic fascia, and this is continued using fingertips, gauze, or a peanut sponge or sponge stick (**Fig. 3**). The dissection is continued to the apex, then inferiorly to the diaphragm, anteriorly to the pericardium, and posteriorly to the spine. This dissection can lead to significant chest-wall bleeding, and in addition to the traditional use of gauze packing, surgeons/ physicians also use transcollation technology (a combination of saline and radiofrequency energy) to create hemostasis with controlled thermal energy during the process. After the parietal pleura has been mobilized, a chest retractor is inserted. Dissection is continued, to separate the pleura from the mediastinum (**Fig. 4**). If the plane between the pericardium and the mediastinal pleura is obliterated, the pericardium may be resected en bloc later during the operation. On the left side, care must be taken to identify the esophagus, the plane between the adventitia of the aorta and the tumor, and the origins of the intercostal vessels. On the right side, care must be taken in dissecting along the superior vena cava. Once the lung and pleura have been mobilized in the upper chest, exposing the hilum, a standard en bloc dissection of the mediastinal lymph nodes is performed, and the specimens are sent to the pathology laboratory for frozen section. At this point, an assessment of all prognostic information (potential completeness of resection, mediastinal lymph node involvement)

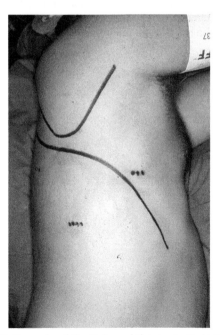

Fig. 1. Example of the S-shaped thoracotomy incision used for extrapleural pneumonectomy. This patient previously had a videothoracoscopy performed (3 incisions also outlined on chest wall). Unfortunately, none of these incisions was placed in a way that they could be incorporated into the thoracotomy incision. (*From* Rusch VW. Technique of extrapleural pneumonectomy for malignant pleural mesothelioma. In: Pearson FG, Patterson A, Cooper J, et al, editors. Pearson's Thoracic & Esophageal Surgery. 3rd edition. New York: Churchill Livingstone; 2008. vol. 97. p. 1187.)

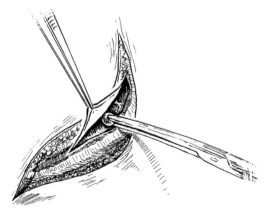

Fig. 2. The extrapleural plane is opened after resection of the sixth rib. (*From* Rusch VW. Technique of extrapleural pneumonectomy for malignant pleural mesothelioma. In: Pearson FG, Patterson A, Cooper J, et al, editors. Pearson's Thoracic & Esophageal Surgery. 3rd edition. New York: Churchill Livingstone; 2008. vol. 97. p. 1188.)

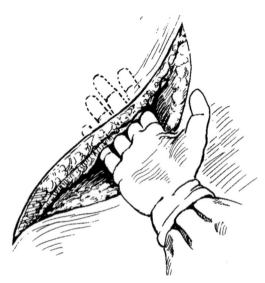

Fig. 3. The parietal pleura is bluntly dissected away from the endothoracic fascia. (*From* Rusch VW. Technique of extrapleural pneumonectomy for malignant pleural mesothelioma. In: Pearson FG, Patterson A, Cooper J, et al, editors. Pearson's Thoracic & Esophageal Surgery. 3rd edition. New York: Churchill Livingstone; 2008. vol. 97. p. 1188.)

contributes to the decision of whether to perform P/D or EPP.

If the decision is made to perform EPP, attention is then turned to resection of the diaphragm. A palpable edge between the tumor and the normal diaphragmatic surface or peritoneum is identified, and this plane is entered, to allow mobilization of the tumor from the posterior costophrenic angle (**Fig. 5**). To provide traction on the diaphragm, the tumor is rotated up into the thoracotomy incision. The depth of dissection, ranging from resection of the entire thickness of the diaphragm (peeling it away from the peritoneum) to superficial dissection into the diaphragmatic muscle (using electrocautery), depends on the extent of invasion. To reduce the risk of intra-abdominal tumor implants, entering the peritoneum should be avoided as much as possible; this is most difficult over the central tendon, but any opening in the peritoneum should be closed immediately. The diaphragmatic portion of the tumor is mobilized back to the pericardium (**Fig. 6**). The hilar structures are divided. In most cases, the mainstem bronchus is transected first, followed by the inferior pulmonary vein, the superior pulmonary vein, and finally the main pulmonary artery. If resection

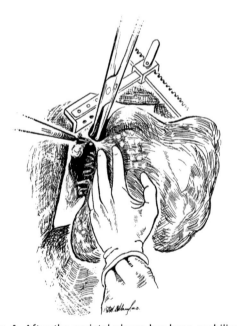

Fig. 4. After the parietal pleura has been mobilized from the chest wall, a chest retractor is inserted, and the mediastinal pleura is freed from the mediastinal structures under direct vision using a combination of sharp and blunt dissection. (*From* Rusch VW. Technique of extrapleural pneumonectomy for malignant pleural mesothelioma. In: Pearson FG, Patterson A, Cooper J, et al, editors. Pearson's Thoracic & Esophageal Surgery. 3rd edition. New York: Churchill Livingstone; 2008. vol. 97. p. 1188.)

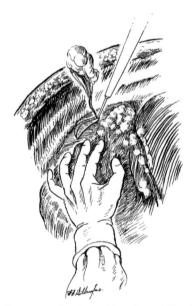

Fig. 5. The tumor has been bluntly mobilized out of the costophrenic sulcus. Strong traction is placed on the pleural tumor and underlying lung, and cautery is used to dissect the diaphragmatic surface of the tumor away from the diaphragmatic muscle or peritoneum. (*From* Rusch VW. Technique of extrapleural pneumonectomy for malignant pleural mesothelioma. In: Pearson FG, Patterson A, Cooper J, et al, editors. Pearson's Thoracic & Esophageal Surgery. 3rd edition. New York: Churchill Livingstone; 2008. vol. 97. p. 1189.)

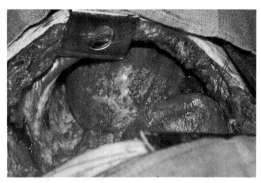

Fig. 6. Intraoperative view of the peritoneum and remaining strands of diaphragmatic muscle after resection of the hemidiaphragm during extrapleural pneumonectomy. The pericardium is also visible in the lower right-hand corner of the photograph. (*From* Rusch VW. Technique of extrapleural pneumonectomy for malignant pleural mesothelioma. In: Pearson FG, Patterson A, Cooper J, et al, editors. Pearson's Thoracic & Esophageal Surgery. 3rd edition. New York: Churchill Livingstone; 2008. vol. 97. p. 1189.)

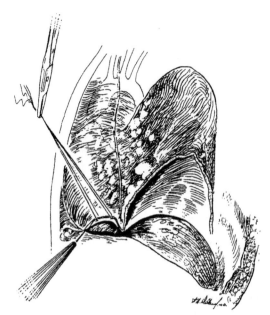

Fig. 7. The pericardium is opened after the tumor has been completely mobilized from all other directions, including the diaphragm. (*From* Rusch VW. Technique of extrapleural pneumonectomy for malignant pleural mesothelioma. In: Pearson FG, Patterson A, Cooper J, et al, editors. Pearson's Thoracic & Esophageal Surgery. 3rd edition. New York: Churchill Livingstone; 2008. vol. 97. p. 1190.)

of the pericardium is required it is performed during this last phase of the operation, as traction on the pericardium can cause arrhythmias and hemodynamic instability. As the hilar structures are dissected out, the pericardium is gradually opened (**Fig. 7**). Traction sutures are placed on the pericardium, to prevent it from retracting to the contralateral side and also to stabilize the position of the heart (**Fig. 8**). The specimen, consisting of the pleura, lung, diaphragm, and occasionally the pericardium, is removed en bloc and sent to the pathology laboratory (**Fig. 9**).

Reconstruction of the diaphragm is then performed, generally with a nonabsorbable material such as polytetrafluoroethylene (Gore-Tex). If the diaphragm has been resected to the costal insertion, the mesh is secured by placing sutures around the ribs laterally and by suturing to the crus posteriorly and to the edge of the pericardium medially (**Fig. 10**). The reconstruction must be strategically positioned at the same level as that of the native diaphragm (tenth intercostal space posteriorly, eighth and ninth intercostal spaces anteriorly and laterally), to avoid complicating the administration of adjuvant radiation therapy, particularly to the posterior costophrenic sulcus. The pericardial defect may be reconstructed with absorbable mesh, to prevent herniation and to maintain the heart's central position, minimizing exposure to subsequent radiation (**Figs. 11** and **12**). A 32F right-angle chest tube is placed over the diaphragmatic reconstruction. The thoracotomy incision is closed, with care taken to reapproximate the intercostal muscles, to ensure a watertight seal and prevent leakage of pleural fluid.

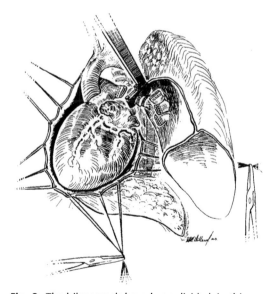

Fig. 8. The hilar vessels have been divided, in this case from within the pericardium. Traction sutures are placed on the edge of the pericardium as it is opened to prevent it from retracting into the contralateral hemithorax. (*From* Rusch VW. Technique of extrapleural pneumonectomy for malignant pleural mesothelioma. In: Pearson FG, Patterson A, Cooper J, et al, editors. Pearson's Thoracic & Esophageal Surgery. 3rd edition. New York: Churchill Livingstone; 2008. vol. 97. p. 1190.)

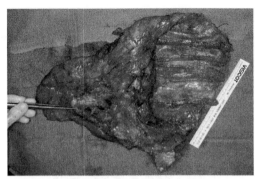

Fig. 9. Example of an extrapleural pneumonectomy specimen with an en bloc removal of the pleura, lung, and portions of the pericardium and hemidiaphragm. The forceps is holding the bronchus. (*From* Rusch VW. Technique of extrapleural pneumonectomy for malignant pleural mesothelioma. In: Pearson FG, Patterson A, Cooper J, et al, editors. Pearson's Thoracic & Esophageal Surgery. 3rd edition. New York: Churchill Livingstone; 2008. vol. 97. p. 1190.)

If P/D is deemed to be the most appropriate procedure, the dissection of the parietal pleura and the tumor continues until complete mobilization of the lung is achieved. In cases where pleura/tumor are inseparable from the pericardium or diaphragm, the involved structures are removed

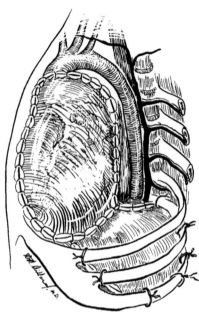

Fig. 11. The completed pericardial and diaphragmatic reconstruction. Laterally, the diaphragm is secured by sutures placed around the ribs. (*From* Rusch VW. Technique of extrapleural pneumonectomy for malignant pleural mesothelioma. In: Pearson FG, Patterson A, Cooper J, et al, editors. Pearson's Thoracic & Esophageal Surgery. 3rd edition. New York: Churchill Livingstone; 2008. vol. 97. p. 1191.)

en bloc and reconstructed, as described for EPP. Once the parietal pleura and lung are completely mobilized, an incision is created through the parietal pleura, tumor, and visceral pleura, to identify

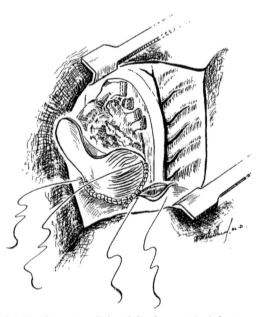

Fig. 10. The pericardial and diaphragmatic defects are reconstructed with prosthetic material. (*From* Rusch VW. Technique of extrapleural pneumonectomy for malignant pleural mesothelioma. In: Pearson FG, Patterson A, Cooper J, et al, editors. Pearson's Thoracic & Esophageal Surgery. 3rd edition. New York: Churchill Livingstone; 2008. vol. 97. p. 1191.)

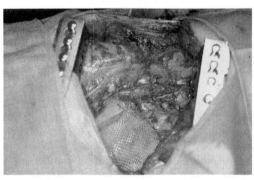

Fig. 12. Intraoperative view of a partially completed pericardial reconstruction using absorbable mesh. The photograph is taken from the anterior aspect of the incision. The esophagus and spine are visible in the upper part of the photograph. (*From* Rusch VW. Technique of extrapleural pneumonectomy for malignant pleural mesothelioma. In: Pearson FG, Patterson A, Cooper J, et al, editors. Pearson's Thoracic & Esophageal Surgery. 3rd edition. New York: Churchill Livingstone; 2008. vol. 97. p. 1191.)

a subtle plane between the visceral pleura and lung parenchyma. Blunt dissection is performed again with fingers, gauze, and a peanut sponge or sponge stick, making sure to achieve a complete resection that includes the visceral pleura and tumor and that extends into the fissures, until the entire visceral pleura, parietal pleura, and tumor are mobilized down to the hilar structures. The specimen is then amputated and sent to the pathology laboratory. After thorough hemostasis is achieved, 4 chest tubes are placed: anteriorly, laterally, angled (preferentially aimed anteriorly), and posteriorly.

Postoperative Care

After P/D the chest tubes are initially placed to suction, to maximize lung expansion and to treat air leaks. During the following postoperative days the tubes are removed as appropriate, depending on fluid output and resolution of air leaks. After EPP the chest tube is placed to gravity drainage for 24 to 72 hours, until drainage becomes sero-sanguinous, to avoid the development of a large hemothorax. To prevent leakage of pleural fluid, a purse-string suture is placed and tied around the chest-tube site after removal of the tube. Supraventricular arrhythmias occur in approximately one-third of patients after EPP; therefore, surgeons/physicians start diltiazem prophylactically on postoperative day 1 and prescribe it for 6 weeks in total. Refractory arrhythmias may occur with mediastinal shift. If this is noted on the chest radiograph, aspiration of the pleural space can be performed, with the patient in the upright position, using a thoracentesis catheter at the first or second intercostal space at the midclavicular line. No more than 500 mL of air and/or fluid should be removed at a time, to avoid too rapid or dramatic a shift of the mediastinum. Other routine aspects of postoperative care after pneumonectomy apply, such as early ambulation, deep venous thrombosis prophylaxis, diligent pulmonary toilet, and careful fluid management, with minimization of intravenous crystalloid solution.

Follow-Up

The initial postoperative visit occurs 2 weeks after discharge, and referral to radiation oncology care should be immediate, to ensure that adjuvant therapy can be initiated within 4 to 6 weeks of the operation. CT imaging of the chest and abdomen is obtained for the planning of radiation treatment, then repeated 1 month after the initiation of adjuvant therapy and then every 4 to 6 months, for the first 2 to 3 years after the operation, after which time imaging is extended to once a year.

SUMMARY

MPM is a difficult disease to treat surgically. The diffuse nature of MPM frequently requires radical resection, which can lead to macroscopic complete resection but is associated with significant morbidity and mortality. Unfortunately, there are no randomized studies to help guide the decision to perform EPP versus P/D when surgical intervention is pursued.

However, significant therapeutic strides, particularly in the form of multimodality therapy, have been made during the last few decades, thanks to a greater understanding of the disease, new chemotherapeutic agents, and improvements in radiation technology. From a surgical standpoint, significant controversy remains regarding the indications for EPP versus P/D when patients are physiologically candidates for both. In the absence of strong evidence-based guidelines, the decision regarding which operation to perform should always take into account the ability to achieve a complete resection, the available adjuvant therapies, and the prognostic factors. Traditionally P/D was performed in patients with minimal disease, and EPP was performed in patients with greater tumor burden. In more recent years, the clinical indications for P/D have expanded to include patients whose findings on surgical exploration suggest a worse prognosis (eg, positive mediastinal lymph node involvement), to spare them the more radical and potentially riskier intervention of EPP. P/D may also become more popular as adjuvant therapies evolve, considering that one of the most convincing advantages of performing EPP at this time is the ability to offer therapeutic doses of radiation therapy, which cannot be administered to patients after P/D. Overall, the treatment of MPM is a complicated and dynamic topic, and patients should be cared for at centers with multidisciplinary expertise.

REFERENCES

1. Centers for Disease Control and Prevention. Malignant mesothelioma mortality—United States, 1999-2005. MMWR Morb Mortal Wkly Rep 2009;58(15):393–6.
2. Centers for Disease Control and Prevention. Work-related lung disease surveillance report 2007. Cincinnati (OH): US Dept of Health and Human Services, CDC, National Institute for Occupational Safety and Health; 2008. Available at: http://www.cdc.gov/niosh/docs/2008-143. Accessed September 1, 2012.
3. Adams RF, Gleeson FV. Percutaneous image-guided cutting-needle biopsy of the pleura in the presence

of a suspected malignant effusion. Radiology 2001;
219:510–4.

4. Boutin C, Rey F. Thoracoscopy in pleural malignant mesothelioma: a prospective study of 188 consecutive patients. Part 1: diagnosis. Cancer 1993;72:389–93.

5. Rusch V, Venkatraman E. The importance of surgical staging in the treatment of malignant pleural mesothelioma. J Thorac Cardiovasc Surg 1996;111:815–26.

6. Flores RM, Routledge T, Seshan VE, et al. The impact of lymph node station on survival in 348 patients with surgically resected malignant pleural mesothelioma: implications for revision of the American Joint Committee on Cancer staging system. J Thorac Cardiovasc Surg 2008;136:605–10.

7. Pass HI, Temeck BK, Kranda K, et al. Preoperative tumor volume is associated with outcome in malignant pleural mesothelioma. J Thorac Cardiovasc Surg 1998;115:310–8.

8. Flores RM, Akhurst T, Gonen M, et al. Positron emission tomography predicts survival in malignant pleural mesothelioma. J Thorac Cardiovasc Surg 2006;132:763–8.

9. Rice D. Surgery for malignant pleural mesothelioma. Ann Diagn Pathol 2009;13(1):65–72.

10. Treasure T, Lang-Lazdunski L, Waller D, et al. Extrapleural pneumonectomy versus no extra-pleural pneumonectomy for patients with malignant pleural mesothelioma: clinical outcomes of the Mesothelioma and Radical Surgery (MARS) randomized feasibility study. Lancet Oncol 2011;12(8):763–72.

11. Flores RM, Pass HI, Seshan VE, et al. Extrapleural pneumonectomy versus pleurectomy/decortications in the surgical management of malignant pleural mesothelioma: results in 663 patients. J Thorac Cardiovasc Surg 2008;135:620–6.

12. Flores RM. Surgical options in malignant pleural mesothelioma: extrapleural pneumonectomy or pleurectomy/decortications. Semin Thorac Cardiovasc Surg 2009;21:149–53.

13. Martin-Ucar AE, Nakas A, Edwards JG, et al. Case-control study between extrapleural pneumonectomy and radical pleurectomy/decortication for pathological N2 malignant pleural mesothelioma. Eur J Cardiothorac Surg 2007;31(5):765–70.

14. Pass HI. Malignant pleural mesothelioma: surgical roles and novel therapies. Clin Lung Cancer 2001; 3(2):102–17.

15. Vogelzang NJ, Rusthoven JJ, Symanowski J, et al. Phase III study of pemetrexed in combination with cisplatin versus cisplatin alone in patients with malignant pleural mesothelioma. J Clin Oncol 2003;21(14):2636–44.

16. Maasilta P. Deterioration in lung function following hemithoracic irradiation for pleural mesothelioma. Int J Radiat Oncol Biol Phys 1991;20:433–8.

17. Gupta V, Mychalczak B, Krug L, et al. Hemithoracic radiation therapy after pleurectomy/decortications

for malignant pleural mesothelioma. Int J Radiat Oncol Biol Phys 2005;63:1045–52.

18. Baldini EH, Recht A, Strauss GM, et al. Patterns of failure after trimodality therapy for malignant pleural mesothelioma. Ann Thorac Surg 1997;63:334–8.

19. Rusch V, Rosenzweig K, Venkatraman E, et al. A phase II trial of surgical resection and adjuvant high-dose hemithoracic radiation for malignant pleural mesothelioma. J Thorac Cardiovasc Surg 2001;122:788–95.

20. Boutin C, Rey F, Viallat JR. Prevention of malignant seeding after invasive diagnostic procedures in patients with pleural mesothelioma: a randomized trial of local radiotherapy. Chest 1995;108:754–8.

21. Weder W, Kestenholz P, Taverna C, et al. Neoadjuvant chemotherapy followed by extrapleural pneumonectomy in malignant pleural mesothelioma. J Clin Oncol 2004;22(17):3451–7.

22. Pagan V, Ceron L, Paccagnella A, et al. 5-year prospective results of trimodality treatment for malignant pleural mesothelioma. J Cardiovasc Surg (Torino) 2006;47(5):595–601.

23. Flores RM, Krug LM, Rosenzweig KE, et al. Induction chemotherapy, extrapleural pneumonectomy, and postoperative high-dose radiotherapy for locally advanced malignant pleural mesothelioma: a phase II trial. J Thorac Oncol 2006;1: 289–95.

24. Weder W, Stahel RA, Bernhard J, et al. Multicenter trial of neo-adjuvant chemotherapy followed by extrapleural pneumonectomy in malignant pleural mesothelioma. Ann Oncol 2007;18(7):1196–202.

25. Rea F, Marulli G, Bortolotti L, et al. Induction chemotherapy, extrapleural pneumonectomy, and adjuvant hemi-thoracic radiation in malignant pleural mesothelioma: feasibility and results. Lung Cancer 2007; 57(1):89–95.

26. Batirel HF, Metintas M, Caglar HB, et al. Trimodality treatment of malignant pleural mesothelioma. J Thorac Oncol 2008;3(5):499–504.

27. Krug LM, Pass HI, Rusch V, et al. Multicenter phase II trial of neoadjuvant pemetrexed plus cisplatin followed by extrapleural pneumonectomy and radiation for malignant pleural mesothelioma. J Clin Oncol 2009;27:3007–13.

28. Bolukbas S, Manegold C, Eberlein M, et al. Survival after trimodality therapy for malignant pleural mesothelioma: radical pleurectomy, chemotherapy with cisplatin/pemetrexed and radiotherapy. Lung Cancer 2011;71(1):75–81.

29. Van Schil PE, Baas P, Gaafar R, et al. Trimodality therapy for malignant pleural mesothelioma: results from an EORTC phase II multicentre trial. Eur Respir J 2010;36(6):1362–9.

30. Zauderer MG, Krug LM. The evolution of multimodality therapy for malignant pleural mesothelioma. Curr Treat Options Oncol 2011;12(2):163–72.

31. Pass HI, Temeck BK, Kranda K, et al. Phase III randomized trial of surgery with or without intraoperative photodynamic therapy and postoperative immuno-chemotherapy for malignant pleural mesothelioma. Ann Surg Oncol 1997;4:628–33.

32. Rusch V, Saltz L, Venkatranam E, et al. A phase II trial of pleurectomy/decortications followed by intra-pleural and systemic chemotherapy for malignant pleural mesothelioma. J Clin Oncol 1994;12(6): 1156–63.

33. Richards WG, Zellos L, Bueno R, et al. Phase I to II study of pleurectomy/decortications and intraoperative intracavitary hyperthermic cisplatin lavage for mesothelioma. J Clin Oncol 2006;24:1561–7.

34. Rosenzweig KE, Zauderer MG, Laser B, et al. Pleural intensity-modulated radiotherapy for malignant pleural mesothelioma. Int J Radiat Oncol Biol Phys 2012;83(4):1278–83.

35. Heelan RT, Rusch V, Begg CB, et al. Staging of malignant pleural mesothelioma: comparison of CT and MR imaging. AJR Am J Roentgenol 1999;172: 1039–47.

36. Flores RM, Akhurst T, Gonen M, et al. Positron emission tomography defines metastatic disease but not locoregional disease in patients with malignant pleural mesothelioma. J Thorac Cardiovasc Surg 2003;126:11–6.

37. Erasmus JJ, Truong MT, Smythe WR, et al. Integrated computed tomography-positron emission tomography in patients with potentially resectable malignant pleural mesothelioma: staging implications. J Thorac Cardiovasc Surg 2005;129(6):1364–70.

38. Rice DC, Erasmus JJ, Stevens CW, et al. Extended surgical staging for potentially resectable malignant pleural mesothelioma. Ann Thorac Surg 2005;80(6): 1988–92.

Hemothorax
Etiology, Diagnosis, and Management

Stephen R. Broderick, MD

KEYWORDS

- Hemothorax • Thoracic • Trauma • Video-assisted thoracic surgery

KEY POINTS

- Initial management of traumatic hemothorax should focus on identification and treatment of life-threatening injuries, control of bleeding, and resuscitation.
- Retained hemothorax is an important entity in the management of the injured patient, as it predisposes to the development of empyema and fibrothorax.
- Early video-assisted thoracic surgery is an effective strategy for the management of retained hemothorax after diagnosis.
- There are multiple causes of spontaneous hemothorax with which the thoracic surgeon should be familiar.

TRAUMATIC HEMOTHORAX

Thoracic trauma continues to be a substantial cause of morbidity and mortality. Chest injuries occur in approximately 60% of multitrauma patients and are responsible for 20% to 25% of trauma-related mortalities. Most thoracic injuries can be managed expectantly with or without tube thoracostomy. An outstanding overview of thoracic trauma in the United States was published in this journal in 2007.[1] A 2004 study of 1359 consecutive patients with chest trauma at a United States level I trauma center demonstrated that only 18% of patients required tube thoracostomy and 2.6% required thoracotomy. In this study, the majority of injuries resulted from a blunt mechanism and the overall mortality was 9.4%.[2] Liman and Colleagues[3] demonstrated a correlation between the number of rib fractures and patient outcomes in a study of 1490 patients following blunt thoracic injury: 6.7% of patients without rib fractures developed hemothorax or pneumothorax, compared with 24.9% of patients with 1 or 2 rib fractures and 81.4% of patients with greater than 2 rib fractures. Tube thoracostomy was required by 17.4% of patients.

Initial Evaluation

Hemothorax should be suspected in any patient arriving at the emergency department following blunt or penetrating thoracic or thoracoabdominal trauma. A high index of suspicion and careful physical examination may prompt appropriate intervention before obtaining imaging studies. Patients with hemodynamic instability or respiratory insufficiency and absent or decreased breath sounds, tracheal deviation, or serious penetrating injuries should have a tube thoracostomy placed as part of initial trauma management.

Imaging

Upright chest radiography is a standard part of trauma evaluation, especially in patients with thoracic trauma. Some clinical situations preclude an upright radiograph, in which case supine films

No funding support was used in the preparation of this article.
The author has nothing to disclose.
Division of Cardiothoracic Surgery, Department of Surgery, Washington University School of Medicine, Campus Box 8234, 660 South Euclid Avenue, St Louis, MO 63110, USA
E-mail address: brodericks@wudosis.wustl.edu

Thorac Surg Clin 23 (2013) 89–96
http://dx.doi.org/10.1016/j.thorsurg.2012.10.003

are acceptable. Blunting of the costophrenic angle or partial or complete opacification of the hemithorax is suggestive of hemothorax. Presence of a small hemothorax may be subtle, as several hundred milliliters of blood can be obscured by the diaphragm and abdominal viscera on upright films. Similarly, in supine patients blood will layer in the pleural space and may appear as little more than haziness in one hemithorax relative to the contralateral side. **Fig. 1** demonstrates haziness of the left lung field on a portable supine chest radiograph obtained during initial trauma evaluation; the patient had a large-volume hemothorax necessitating exploration and repair of the subclavian artery. A large hemothorax may opacify an entire hemithorax or cause mediastinal shift and tension physiology. These findings require immediate intervention.

Computed tomography (CT) has become commonplace in the evaluation of the injured patient, and allows for detection of much smaller amounts of fluid than chest radiography. Fluid in the pleural space is assumed to be blood until proved otherwise. If the nature of fluid in the pleural space is in question (ie, in the case of chronic pleural effusion), measurement of Hounsfield units may prove useful. An arterial blush identified on CT indicates ongoing bleeding and is an indication for urgent intervention (**Fig. 2**). Persistent abnormalities on chest radiographs should be further evaluated by CT, especially in patients who are failing to progress (**Fig. 3**).

In the past decade the use of ultrasonography has become a mainstay in emergency department and trauma evaluation. Ultrasonography is often more readily attainable than CT and can be used in patients who are not stable enough for transport. A prospective study of the utility of ultrasonography in diagnosing hemothorax in 61 trauma patients demonstrated sensitivity of 92% and specificity of 100%. In most cases the ultrasonography result was available to the trauma team before the CT results.[4]

Management

Tube thoracostomy is the first-line treatment of most hemothoraces. Appropriate placement of the tube is critical for effective drainage of the pleural space. Placement should be directed posteriorly to allow for dependent drainage in the supine patient. A thoracostomy tube can be safely placed in the sixth or seventh intercostal space at the mid-axillary line in most patients by an experienced operator. Historically, larger-diameter chest tubes have been used for suspected hemothorax to prevent clotted blood from obstructing drainage. The Advanced Trauma Life Support protocol calls for use of a 36F chest tube in educational materials.[5] However, a recent prospective analysis of size 28F to 32F tubes compared with 36F to 40F tubes in 293 patients at a level I trauma center demonstrated no difference in outcomes based on size of chest tube placed.[6] Most surgeons place 32F or 36F tubes for suspected hemothorax. When feasible, patients should receive antimicrobial prophylaxis with cefazolin before tube thoracostomy. This recommendation is an advisory of a working group of the Eastern Association for Surgery for Trauma.[7]

Traditional indications for surgical intervention in acute traumatic hemothorax include initial drainage of more than 1500 mL following tube thoracostomy or drainage of more than 200 mL per hour for 4 hours. However, the physiologic parameters and overall condition of the patient must be the primary driver for surgical intervention, rather than absolute volume of initial or ongoing chest-tube output.

The surgical approach to acute thoracic traumatic injury is tailored to the suspected injury and clinical situation. The standard initial approach to traumatic hemothorax is the anterior thoracotomy. Performed through the fourth interspace, this approach allows for rapid assessment of intrathoracic injuries and temporary hemostasis as necessary. A right anterior thoracotomy allows for access to the right atrium, superior vena cava, right lung, right pulmonary hilum, and ascending aorta. Left anterior thoracotomy provides access to the left and right ventricles, pulmonary artery, and left pulmonary hilum. This approach also provides access for release of

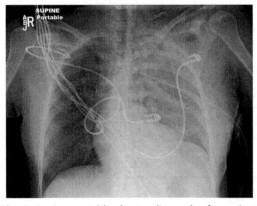

Fig. 1. Supine portable chest radiograph of a patient obtained during initial trauma evaluation. A large volume of blood in the pleural space may appear as haziness as blood layers posteriorly. The CT scan of this same patient is presented in **Fig. 2**.

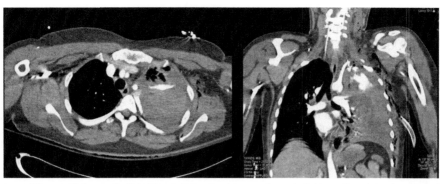

Fig. 2. Contrast CT scan of the patient in **Fig. 1**. Note the large-volume left hemothorax and contrast blush, indicating need for immediate intervention. This patient had an injury to the left subclavian artery and vein.

pericardial tamponade and clamping of the descending aorta for temporary control of intraabdominal hemorrhage. The anterior thoracotomy can be extended in a variety of ways to provide additional access. Extension across the sternum creates a "clamshell" incision and provides excellent access to mediastinal structures. Addition of median sternotomy allows for better access to the heart and structures in the superior mediastinum. Cervical or supraclavicular incisions are useful adjuncts to provide access to arch vessels or injuries to cervical or subclavian vessels. The anterior thoracotomy can also be extended to a thoracoabdominal approach for combined thoracic and abdominal injuries.[8]

Median sternotomy is the preferred approach to isolated injuries to the heart, great vessels, or aortic arch. Sternotomy may take longer to perform for surgeons not facile with the technique or if proper equipment is not immediately available. Postoperative morbidity associated with sternal nonunion or osteomyelitis may be higher in the trauma setting in comparison with elective sternotomy. Posterolateral thoracotomy provides excellent access to the ipsilateral lung, hilum, and pleural space as well as the posterior mediastinum. It is the preferred approach for most esophageal injuries, airway injuries, or pulmonary resections when necessary. Posterolateral thoracotomy should, however, be reserved for stable patients because patient positioning limits access to the contralateral pleural space or abdomen. The lateral decubitus position also predisposes patients to contamination of the opposite lung with airway secretions or blood. The use of video-assisted thoracic surgery (VATS) in the acute trauma setting is controversial. VATS may be useful to explore the pleural space, control minor bleeding, or evacuate hemothorax. Its use, however, should be reserved for experienced operators and limited indications.

RETAINED HEMOTHORAX

Whereas initial tube thoracostomy may effectively drain liquid blood from the pleural space, clotted

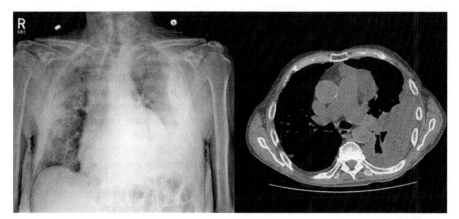

Fig. 3. Persistent abnormalities on chest radiographs should be evaluated by CT to assess for retained hemothorax. In this patient hemothorax developed gradually following blunt chest injury.

or loculated collections of blood may not be evacuated by single or even multiple chest tubes. Retained blood in the pleural space is a risk factor for the development of further complications including empyema[9–11] and fibrothorax. The diagnosis and management of retained hemothorax after thoracic trauma remains controversial and has been the subject of several recent investigations in the trauma literature, including a prospective multicenter analysis undertaken by the American Association for the Surgery of Trauma (AAST).[12]

The presence of retained hemothorax may not be readily apparent on routine radiographs. Suspicion of inadequate drainage should prompt evaluation by CT imaging. Observation is an acceptable strategy for small collections.[13] The AAST prospective study found that 30.8% of patients with retained hemothorax after initial trauma intervention were managed by observation alone. Of these patients, 82.2% required no further interventions. On multivariate analysis, clinical predictors of successful observation were initial chest-tube indication of pneumothorax and CT estimated volume of hemothorax of less than 300 mL.[12]

Insertion of a second thoracostomy tube or, more recently, the use of image-guided drainage is another approach to draining retained hemothoraces. These approaches are unlikely to be successful in adequately draining loculated or clotted collections. A randomized prospective trial by Meyer and colleagues[14] compared the use of additional chest-tube placement with thoracoscopy for evacuation of retained hemothorax after initial chest-tube placement. The thoracoscopy group demonstrated a shorter duration of chest-tube drainage (2.53 vs 4.50 days, $P<.02$), shorter hospital stay (5.40 vs 8.13 days, $P<.02$), and reduced total hospital costs. Furthermore, in the 2012 AAST prospective trial 64% of patients in whom an additional chest tube was placed required subsequent intervention for retained hemothorax; 41% of patients undergoing image-guided drainage required subsequent interventions.[12]

The use of fibrinolytic therapy administered through an indwelling chest tube has been extensively studied for empyema and parapneumonic effusion, for which it has been shown to decrease the frequency of surgical intervention.[15] The utility of this modality for retained hemothorax in trauma patients is less evident. Multiple studies in trauma patients have demonstrated that fibrinolytic therapy can result in effective drainage of the pleural space.[16–19] However, analysis of these results are plagued by small sample sizes, lack of controls, and difficulty in quantifying resolution of hemothorax.[16] A retrospective comparison of patients treated with intrapleural streptokinase or thoracoscopy for the management of retained hemothorax showed a shorter hospital stay and less frequent need for thoracotomy in the thoracoscopy group.[20] Although a prospective comparison with thoracoscopy is lacking, fibrinolytic therapy may serve as a useful adjunct to initial chest-tube drainage or as an alternative to surgical intervention in patients deemed unfit for more invasive procedures.

Several studies over the past decade have demonstrated the effectiveness of VATS for the management of retained traumatic hemothorax.[15,21,22] The visualization afforded by VATS allows for thorough inspection and evacuation of the pleural space, and accurate placement of drains to allow for ongoing drainage as necessary. VATS was the most common initial management approach after diagnosis of retained hemothorax in the 2012 AAST study, and patients managed by VATS required no further therapy in 70% of cases.[12] The timing of VATS in patients with retained hemothorax is a matter of debate. However, it appears that early intervention is generally more successful and less frequently requires conversion to thoracotomy.[22–24]

Despite its associated morbidity, thoracotomy remains the approach with which the effectiveness of other interventions must be compared. Thoracotomy proved the most effective means by which to treat retained hemothorax in the 2012 AAST prospective study, with 79% of patients requiring no further intervention. Factors that predicted eventual need for thoracotomy included associated diaphragmatic injury and failure to administer antibiotics at the time of initial chest-tube placement.[12]

Retained hemothorax puts patients at risk for development of empyema. A recent study of 328 trauma patients with retained hemothorax from 20 centers demonstrated an overall incidence of empyema of 26.8%. Risk factors for the development of empyema included rib fractures, injury severity score (ISS) greater than 25, or the need for additional procedures to address retained hemothorax. Of patients developing empyema after retained hemothorax, 94.3% required additional interventions, with many requiring 2 or more interventions beyond initial chest-tube insertion. After adjusting for the baseline characteristics, patients who developed empyema after retained hemothorax had significantly prolonged stays in the intensive care unit and hospital in comparison with those who did not.[11]

SPONTANEOUS HEMOTHORAX

It is important to distinguish between hemorrhagic effusion and hemothorax. The hematocrit of any bloody effusion should be measured to rule out hemothorax. Pleural fluid will appear similar to blood with a hematocrit as low as 5%. Hemothorax is defined as pleural fluid with a hematocrit greater than 50% of the patient's blood hematocrit, although hematocrit may be somewhat lower in patients with long-standing hemothoraces. Most cases of hemothorax result from thoracic trauma or invasive thoracic procedures such as thoracentesis or placement of a vascular catheter. However, there is a variety of clinical entities other than trauma that can result in the accumulation of blood in the pleural space (**Box 1**). The data regarding spontaneous hemothorax is limited to case reports and series. The major entities with which the thoracic surgeon should be familiar are reviewed here.

Spontaneous Hemopneumothorax

Approximately 5% of patients who present with spontaneous pneumothorax will have concomitant hemothorax. The amount of blood in the pleural space can vary from several hundred milliliters to more than 1.5 L, and presentation may range from asymptomatic to hemorrhagic shock.[25] The source of bleeding in spontaneous hemopneumothorax is variable, but most commonly results from tearing of vascularized adhesions between the parietal and visceral pleura. The presence of a pneumothorax prevents tamponade from the lung and allows blood under systemic pressure to accumulate in the pleural space.

Management of spontaneous hemopneumothorax consists of tube thoracostomy to allow for drainage of the hemothorax and reexpansion of the lung. Subsequent management is not standardized. In a review of 71 patients with spontaneous hemopneumothorax by Kakaris and Colleagues,[26] conservative treatment was effective in 22.5% of cases; 39% of patients were in shock at presentation and were taken for immediate surgery; and the remaining patients had surgery on an elective basis for hemostasis, hemothorax evacuation, and resection of bullae. In the author's opinion, early VATS is the preferred strategy for patients with spontaneous hemopneumothorax, as it allows for thorough inspection of the pleural space, control of any ongoing bleeding, and evacuation of the hemothorax. VATS also allows the surgeon to properly address the etiology of the pneumothorax. However, in a patient with a small hemothorax (<300 mL), stable hemodynamics and fully inflated lung after chest-tube insertion observation is not unreasonable.

Vascular Etiology

Aortic dissection or rupture of thoracic aortic aneurysms is a major vascular cause of hemothorax. These entities generally present with chest pain, and the aortic abnormality is evident on contrast CT scan of the chest. Detailed discussion of the management of these entities is beyond the scope of this review.

Type IV Ehlers-Danlos syndrome occurs when a defect in the production of type III collagen results in thin-walled, ectatic vessels susceptible to aneurysmal dilation and rupture. Hemothorax has resulted in this disease from spontaneous rupture of the internal mammary artery, pulmonary arterial bleeding, or ruptured bullae.[27–29]

Pulmonary arteriovenous malformations (AVMs) are a rare entity usually associated with hereditary hemorrhagic telangiectasia (HHT; also known as Osler-Weber-Rendu syndrome). These lesions consist of abnormal communication between the pulmonary arterial and venous circulations, and are usually congenital.[30] HHT is transmitted in an autosomal dominant fashion and results in AVMs of the skin, mucous membranes, and visceral organs. Pulmonary AVMs vary from microscopic to several centimeters in size, and can be found in the pulmonary parenchyma as well as on the pleural surface. Patients with

---

Box 1
Common causes of spontaneous hemothorax

Spontaneous hemopneumothorax

Vascular

    Aortic dissection/aneurysm

    Arteriovenous malformations

    Aneurysmal disease (Ehlers-Danlos)

Coagulopathy

    Drug-induced

    Congenital

Neoplastic

    Neurofibromatosis

    Metastatic disease

    Germ cell tumor

    Thymoma

Miscellaneous

    Exostoses

    Endometriosis

multiple or large AVMs are often symptomatic, presenting with shortness of breath or hypoxemia. Rupture of subpleural AVMs can result in hemothorax, whereas parenchymal AVMs may produce hemoptysis. In a series of 143 patients with pulmonary AVM, 5 developed hemothorax.[31] There are reports of more than 30 cases in the literature whereby rupture of pulmonary AVMs caused hemothorax. Over one-third of these cases occurred in the later stages of pregnancy as blood volume and cardiac output increase substantially.[31–33] Treatment of hemothorax related to pulmonary AVMs consists initially of drainage of the pleural space. In stable patients with a slow rate of bleeding, embolization of the AVM may be pursued. However, additional AVMs, recanalization, and development of collateral vessels may occur in the future. Patients with hemodynamic instability or rapid rate of bleeding should be managed with immediate surgery, preferably by a VATS approach.

Costal Exostoses

Costal exostoses represent a rare cause of spontaneous hemothorax or hemopneumothorax. These bony outgrowths from the ribs may be solitary or multiple, as in the hereditary multiple exostoses syndrome. There are many cases reported in the literature in which exostoses result in hemothorax. The exact mechanism of bleeding is unclear, but is thought to be due to injury to the visceral pleura and underlying pulmonary parenchyma from direct contact with relatively sharp exostoses. Alternatively, bleeding may result from rupture of dilated vessels associated with repetitive irritation of the visceral pleura.[29,34,35] Management consists of control of bleeding, evacuation of the hemothorax, and resection of exostoses to prevent future episodes.

Endometriosis

Spontaneous hemothorax or hemopneumothorax may result from endometrial implants on the pleural surface and their response to cyclical hormonal changes in menstruating women. Endometrial implantation occurs as a result of migration of endometrial tissue across fenestrations in the diaphragm. Known as catamenial hemothorax, this entity is usually managed by hormonal therapy designed to limit estrogen secretion or produce amenorrhea. In the event of failure of hormonal therapy or recurrent episodes, exploration of the pleural space and resection of endometrial implants may be necessary.[36,37]

Neoplasia

Several neoplastic processes may result in the accumulation of blood in the pleural space. Advanced lung cancer frequently results in development of malignant effusions, but is rarely the cause of hemothorax. Neurofibromatosis (von Recklinghausen disease) has frequently resulted in hemothorax either by invasion of vascular structures by neurofibroma or as a result of arterial dysplasia.[29,38–40] Metastatic spread of sarcomas to the lung, particularly angiosarcoma, is a frequent cause of hemothorax associated with malignancy.[41] This entity portends a poor prognosis, with an 8-month mortality rate of greater than 80%.[29] Hepatocellular carcinoma is another malignancy associated with metastatic spread to the lungs and subsequent hemothorax.[42] Finally, primary mediastinal tumors such as thymoma or germ cell tumors have been reported to rupture into the pleural space, resulting in hemothorax.[43,44]

Coagulopathy

Hemothorax may occur with the administration of anticoagulant therapy for multiple indications. Blood may accumulate either spontaneously or as a result of minimal trauma in patients with abnormal coagulation parameters. Many cases of anticoagulation-associated hemothorax have been documented in the literature, most commonly in the setting of treatment of pulmonary embolic disease. Bleeding may also occur with the administration of systemic or intrapleural thrombolytics or in the setting of inherited coagulation disorders such as hemophilia.[45,46] Regardless of the underlying condition, the mainstay of therapy is correction of the coagulopathy followed by evacuation of the hemothorax. Bleeding is usually self-limited once coagulopathy is corrected.

SUMMARY

This article reviews the major causes and management of hemothorax. Most hemothoraces are the result of blunt or penetrating thoracic trauma. Initial management is focused on identification and treatment of life-threatening injuries, control of bleeding, and resuscitation. In many cases acute hemothorax can be addressed with tube thoracostomy alone. Retained hemothorax is an important entity in the management of the injured patient, as it predisposes to the development of empyema and fibrothorax. Though less common, spontaneous hemothorax does occur with some regularity, and the thoracic surgeon should be familiar with its multiple causes and management.

REFERENCES

1. Khandahar SJ, Johnson SB, Calhoon JH. Overview of thoracic trauma in the United States. Thorac Surg Clin 2007;17(1):1–9.
2. Kulshrestha P, Munshi I, Wait R. Profile of chest trauma in a level I trauma center. J Trauma 2004; 57:576–81.
3. Liman ST, Kuzucu A, Irfan A, et al. Chest injury due to blunt trauma. Eur J Cardiothorac Surg 2003;23: 374–8.
4. Brooks A, Davies B, Sethhurst M, et al. Emergency ultrasound in the acute assessment of haemothorax. Emerg Med J 2004;21:44–6.
5. American College of Surgeons. Committee on trauma. ATLS: advanced trauma life support for doctors. 8th edition. Chicago: American College of Surgeons; 2008.
6. Inaba K, Lustenberger T, Recinos G, et al. Does size matter? A prospective analysis of 28-32 versus 36-40 French chest tube size in trauma. J Trauma 2012;72:422–7.
7. Luchette FA, Barie PS, Oswanski MF, et al. Practice management guidelines for prophylactic antibiotic use in tube thoracostomy for traumatic hemopneumothorax: the EAST practice management guideline working group. J Trauma 2000;484:753–7.
8. Losso LC, Ghefter MC. Penetrating thoracic trauma. In: Patterson GA, editor. Pearson's thoracic and esophageal surgery. 3rd edition. Philadelphia: Churchill Livingstone; 2008. p. 1782–5.
9. Eren S, Esme H, Sehitogullari A, et al. The risk factors and management of posttraumatic empyema in trauma patients. Injury 2008;39(1):44–9.
10. Karmy-Jones R, Holevar M, Sullivan RJ, et al. Residual hemothorax after chest tube placement correlates with increased risk of empyema following traumatic injury. Can Respir J 2008;15(5):255–8.
11. DuBose J, Inaba K, Okoye O, et al. Development of posttraumatic empyema in patients with retained hemothorax: results of a prospective, observational AAST study. J Trauma Acute Care Surg 2012;73: 752–7.
12. DuBose J, Inaba K, Demetriades D, et al. Management of post-traumatic retained hemothorax: a prospective, observational, multicenter AAST study. J Trauma Acute Care Surg 2012;72(1):11–22.
13. Bilello JF, Davis JW, Lemaster DM. Occult traumatic hemothorax: when can sleeping dogs lie? Am J Surg 2005;190:844–8.
14. Meyer DM, Jessen ME, Wait MA, et al. Early evacuation of traumatic retained hemothoraces using thoracoscopy: a prospective, randomized trial. Ann Thorac Surg 1997;64(5):1396–400.
15. Cameron R, Davies HR. Intra-pleural fibrinolytic therapy versus conservative management in the treatment of adult parapneumonic effusions and empyema. Cochrane Database Syst Rev 2008;(2):CD002312.
16. Hunt I, Thakar C, Southon R, et al. Establishing a role for intra-pleural fibrinolysis in managing traumatic haemothraces. Interact Cardiovasc Thorac Surg 2009;8:129–33.
17. Kimbrell BJ, Yamzon J, Petrone P, et al. Intrapleural thrombolysis for the management of undrained traumatic hemothorax: a prospective observational study. J Trauma 2007;62:1175–9.
18. Inci I, Ozcelic C, Ulkii R, et al. Intrapleural fibrinolytic treatment of traumatic clotted hemothorax. Chest 1998;1:160–5.
19. Aye RW, Froese DP, Hill LD. Use of purified streptokinase in empyema and hemothorax. Am J Surg 1991;161:560–2.
20. Ogzkaya Y, Akcali M, Bilgin M. Videothoracoscopy versus intrapleural streptokinase for management of undrained traumatic hemothorax: a retrospective study of 65 cases. Injury 2005;36:526–9.
21. Navsaria PH, Vogel RJ, Nicol AJ. Thoracoscopic evacuation of retained posttraumatic hemothorax. Ann Thorac Surg 2004;78:282–5.
22. Velmahos GC, Demetriades D. Early thoracoscopy for the evacuation of undrained haemothorax. Eur J Surg 1999;165:924–9.
23. Morales Uribe CH, Villegas Lanau MI, Petro Sanchez RD. Best timing for thoracoscopic evacuation or retained post-traumatic hemothorax. Surg Endosc 2008;22:91–5.
24. Smith JW, Franklin GA, Harbrecht BG, et al. Early VATS for blunt chest trauma: a management technique underutilized by acute care surgeons. J Trauma 2011;71(1):102–5.
25. Hsu NY, Shis CS, Hsu CP, et al. Spontaneous hemopneumothorax revisited: clinical approach and systemic review of the literature. Ann Thorac Surg 2005;80:1859–63.
26. Kakaris S, Athanassiadi K, Vassilikos K, et al. Spontaneous hemopneumothorax: a rare but life-threatening entity. Eur J Cardiothorac Surg 2004; 25:856–8.
27. Phan TG, Sakulsaengprapha A, Wilson M, et al. Ruptured internal mammary artery aneurysm presenting as massive spontaneous haemothorax in a patient with Ehlers-Danlos syndrome. Aust N Z J Med 1998;28:210–1.
28. Hasan RI, Krysiak P, Deiranyia AK, et al. Spontaneous rupture of the internal mammary artery in Ehlers-Danlos syndrome. J Thorac Cardiovasc Surg 1993;106:184–5.
29. Ali HA, Lippmann M, Mundathaje U, et al. Spontaneous hemothorax: a comprehensive review. Chest 2008;134:1056–65.
30. Gossage JR, Kanj G. Pulmonary arteriovenous malformations: a state of the art review. Am J Respir Crit Care Med 1998;158(2):643–61.

31. Ference BA, Shannon TM, White RI, et al. Life-threatening pulmonary hemorrhage with pulmonary arteriovenous malformations and hereditary hemorrhagic telangiectasia. Chest 1994;106:1387–90.

32. Martinez FJ, Villaneuna AG, Pickering R, et al. Spontaneous hemothorax: report of six cases and review of the literature. Medicine 1992;71:354–68.

33. Esplin MS, Varner MW. Progression of pulmonary arteriovenous malformation during pregnancy: case report and review of the literature. Obstet Gynecol Surv 1997;52:248–53.

34. Bini A, Gazia M, Stella F, et al. Acute massive haemopneumothorax due to solitary costal exostosis. Interact Cardiovasc Thorac Surg 2003;2(4):614–5.

35. Uchida K, Kurihara Y, Sekiguchi S, et al. Spontaneous haemothorax caused by costal exostosis. Eur Respir J 1997;10(3):735–6.

36. Joseph J, Sahn SA. Thoracic endometriosis syndrome: new observations from an analysis of 110 cases. Am J Med 1996;100:164–70.

37. Bagan P, Le Pimpec Barthes F, Assouad J, et al. Catamenial pneumothorax: retrospective study of surgical treatment. Ann Thorac Surg 2003;75:378–81.

38. Miura H, Taira O, Uchida O, et al. Spontaneous haemothorax associate with Von Recklinghausen's disease: review of occurrence in Japan. Thorax 1997;52:577–8.

39. Yoshida K, Tobe S. Dissection and rupture of the left subclavian artery presenting as hemothorax in a patient with Von Recklinghausen's disease. Jpn J Thorac Cardiovasc Surg 2005;53:117–9.

40. Tatebe S, Asami F, Shinohara H, et al. Ruptured aneurysm of the subclavian artery in a patient with von Recklinghausen's disease. Circ J 2005;69:503–6.

41. Liu SF, Wu CC, Lai YF, et al. Massive hemoptysis and hemothorax caused by pleuropulmonary angiosarcoma. Am J Emerg Med 2002;20:374–5.

42. Sohara N, Takagi H, Yamada T, et al. Hepatocellular carcinoma complicated by hemothorax. J Gastroenterol 2000;35:240–4.

43. Caplin JL, Gullan RW, Dymond DS, et al. Hemothorax due to rupture of a benign thymoma. Jpn Heart J 1985;26:123–5.

44. Yang WM, Chen ML, Lin TS. Traumatic hemothorax resulting from rupture of a mediastinal teratoma: a case report. Int Surg 2005;90:241–4.

45. Hsiao CW, Lee SC, Chen JC, et al. Massive spontaneous haemopneumothorax in a patient with haemophilia. ANZ J Surg 2001;71:770–1.

46. Morecroft JA, Lea RE. Haemothorax: a complication of anticoagulation for suspected pulmonary embolism. Br J Clin Pract 1988;42:217–8.

Index

Note: Page numbers of article titles are in **boldface** type.

A

ADA. See *Adenosine deaminase.*
Adenosine deaminase
    in pleural fluid, 7
Anatomy and pathophysiology of the pleura and
    pleural space, **1–10**
Antibiotics
    and empyema, 30
    and parapneumonic effusions, 30
Arteriovenous malformations
    and spontaneous hemothorax, 93, 94
Asbestos
    and malignant mesothelioma, 73, 74, 80
AVM. See *Arteriovenous malformations.*

B

BAPE. See *Benign asbestos pleural effusion.*
Benign asbestos pleural effusion, 38

C

Causes and management of common benign pleural
    effusions, **25–42**
Chemotherapy
    and malignant mesothelioma, 77, 78
Chest radiography
    and pleural effusions, 4, 5
    and trapped lung, 52
CHF. See *Congestive heart failure.*
Cholesterol
    in pleural fluid, 7
Chylothorax
    causes of, 37
    and clinical manifestations, 37
    and exudative pleural effusions, 36–38
    management of, 37, 38
    pathophysiology of, 36, 37
    and pleural effusions, 9
Coagulopathy
    and spontaneous hemothorax, 94
Community-acquired pleural infections
    bacteriology of, 30
Complications
    of large bore vs. small-bore chest tubes, 21, 22
Computed tomography
    and pleural effusions, 5
    and trapped lung, 52
Congestive heart failure

    and clinical manifestations, 27, 28
    management of, 28
    pathophysiology of, 27
    and transudative pleural effusions, 26–28
Connective tissue diseases
    and exudative pleural effusions, 34
Cost
    of large-bore vs. small-bore chest tubes, 22
Costal exostoses
    and spontaneous hemothorax, 94

D

Decision making and algorithm for the management
    of pleural effusions, **11–16**
Decortication
    and malignant pleural effusions, 48, 57, 58
Drug-induced pleural effusions
    and clinical presentation, 33, 34
    management of, 34
    pathophysiology of, 33

E

Effectiveness
    of large-bore vs. small-bore chest tubes, 22
Empyema
    and antibiotics, 30
    bacteriology of, 29
    and drainage, 30, 31
    and exudative pleural effusions, 29–31
    and hemothorax, 36
    and hepatic hydrothorax, 28
    and malignant pleural effusions, 16
    management of, 29
    pathophysiology of, 29
    and pleural effusions, 8
    and rheumatoid arthritis, 34
    and trapped lung, 51–59
Empyema thoracis
    and trapped lung, 52
Empyemectomy
    and trapped lung, 53, 54
Endometriosis
    and spontaneous hemothorax, 94
Eosinophilia
    and pleural fluid, 8
EPP. See *Extrapleural pneumonectomy.*
Extrapleural pneumonectomy
    and malignant mesothelioma, 75–85

http://dx.doi.org/10.1016/S1547-4127(12)00090-4
1547-4127/13/$ – see front matter © 2013 Elsevier Inc. All rights reserved.

Printed and bound by CPI Group (UK) Ltd, Croydon, CR0 4YY

03/10/2024

01040346-0006